KT-420-304

WITHDRAWN FROM
BROMLEY LIBRARIES

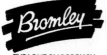

THE
DOS AND
DON'TS

OF
PREGNANCY

Louise Baty

Vie is an imprint of Summersdale Publishers Ltd

Summersdale Publishers Ltd
46 West Street
Chichester
West Sussex
PO19 1RP
UK

www.summersdale.com

Printed and bound in the Czech Republic

ISBN: 978-1-84953-762-9

Substantial discounts on bulk quantities of Summersdale books are available to corporations, professional associations and other organisations. For details contact Nicky Douglas by telephone: +44 (0) 1243 756902, fax: +44 (0) 1243 786300 or email: nicky@summersdale.com.

CONTENTS

Chapter 6 – The Dos and Don'ts for
Preparing for Giving Birth.....................................127

Chapter 7 – Possible Health Problems during Pregnancy....157

INTRODUCTION

Welcome to *The Dos and Don'ts of Pregnancy*!

If you're reading this book because you're already pregnant or are planning on starting a family, congratulations!

This may be your first pregnancy or you might have done it all before. Whatever your situation, pregnancy can be a magical time, filled with excitement, joy and hope for the future.

But the 40 weeks of pregnancy can also be tough – physically, mentally and emotionally.

Although some women revel in their new state, finding themselves full of energy and *joie de vivre*, others never experience the much-talked-about 'bloom' of pregnancy. There may be unpleasant physical hurdles such as morning sickness, exhaustion and heartburn to overcome.

Being an expectant mum, your whole world is shifting on its axis. As your body changes with each passing week, you'll have your own worries to contend with, along with those of your partner.

But, by now, you might have realised something. The most aggravating aspect of being pregnant isn't piles or stretch marks. *It's all the conflicting advice you receive.*

This advice may come from anyone – relatives, friends or even complete strangers. It's usually well meaning and designed to be helpful. But, unfortunately, it can sometimes be unsettling and annoying.

Then there are the seemingly endless and ever-changing lists of official guidelines for having a safe, healthy pregnancy. If you find yourself utterly flummoxed by them all, you're not alone.

In fact, as you embark on this life-changing experience, you may find your mind whirring with questions…

▶ *What is safe to eat and what should I eat?*

▶ *How do I deal with morning sickness?*

▶ *What are my rights at work?*

▶ *Is it normal to feel this exhausted?*

▶ *Can I drink alcohol?*

▶ *Should I exercise?*

▶ *Can sex during pregnancy harm the baby?*

▶ *How do I plan for the birth?*

Knowledge is power. That's why this guide aims to dispel myths and banish confusion by laying out all the current official guidelines, with handy tips and advice from medical experts.

We'll tell you what's happening to your baby at each stage, along with what to expect when it comes to changes in your body.

We've included comments from other parents-to-be who have been exactly where you are now. With a simple layout and chapters dealing with specific trimesters, the book is designed for you to dip into whenever you have a question.

You may prefer to read up on each trimester as you're nearing that stage but if you're looking for a particular point, you can look it up in the index at the back of the book. We've also included a chapter on possible health complications that may arise during pregnancy.

The information is also aimed to help and inform your partner, who may have their own questions.

Every point has been guided by official NHS advice, and we have consulted medical experts for accuracy. However, if you have a real concern about your health or pregnancy, you should consult your GP or midwife.

The main thing to remember: No one knows your body as well as you do. It's your pregnancy and your baby.

In the distant past, women talked in hushed tones about their 'confinement'. Times have changed. Pregnant women carry on working, travelling and enjoying life throughout. So try not to wrap yourself in cotton wool.

Yes, you want to protect yourself and your baby, but following your instincts and using common sense is an essential part of parenthood. There's no better time to start trusting yourself than now.

Above all, enjoy this exciting journey… and good luck!

CHAPTER 1

THE DOs AND DON'Ts FOR DIETARY HEALTH PRE-PREGNANCY AND FOR THE WHOLE NINE MONTHS

Deciding to try for a baby is one of the biggest decisions you will ever make – and certainly the most life changing.

As you're reading this book, it's likely that you want to know how to have a safe, healthy and happy pregnancy. Well, you've come to the right place!

It's good to plan ahead, if you can. So here are some useful tips to put into practice before you even conceive.

Prepare yourself

You should view the months before you conceive as being equally important as the ones during your pregnancy. So it's beneficial to prepare your body before you attempt to conceive your baby.

Adopt a healthier lifestyle – Try to adopt a healthy lifestyle at least 12 months before you try to conceive by:

✓ cutting down your alcohol intake

✓ cutting out recreational drugs

✓ eating a balanced healthy diet (see details in next section)

✓ taking regular exercise

✓ reaching a healthy BMI before conception – this is considered to be between 18.5 and 24.9. (For more details, see page 13.)

✓ stopping smoking

✓ getting plenty of sleep

✓ taking folic acid – around three months before you decide to start trying for a baby, start taking 400 mcg of folic acid each day. (For the reasons why, see page 14 in this chapter.)

Get your finances in order – There's no two ways about it – babies are expensive! It's a good idea to have a financial plan for your maternity leave, if you're going to take it. And it's beneficial to make sure your partner is working to the same plan if possible. If you can start saving money each month before you even start trying for your baby, do.

> ### *Ask your partner for support*
> It's easier to make plans and stick to a healthy lifestyle if your other half is by your side. Try to encourage a healthy parenting partnership by exercising and eating well together. It will stand you in good stead in the long run if you're working together to prepare yourselves for the next stage... parenthood!

General dos and don'ts during pregnancy

Pregnancy is an exciting journey but it's important to know the 'basics' for navigating your way smoothly and safely through each stage. In the following chapters, we'll focus on individual trimesters. But for now, here are some useful general tips for your entire pregnancy.

Look into antenatal care – It's a good idea to know about the antenatal care you're eligible for, as soon as you know you're pregnant.

Meet the professionals – Over the next few months, you will have a series of appointments with medical professionals, whose job it is to look after you and your unborn baby during your pregnancy. Appointments may be with a midwife, your GP or a specialist doctor called an obstetrician.

Tip

If you have any concerns, speak to your midwife or GP

Your midwife or GP should also be your first port of call, if you have any questions or concerns over your pregnancy.

Find out about classes – You may also be offered antenatal classes, so you can find out about the process of pregnancy, labour and possibly also breastfeeding. Your place should be booked in advance and your midwife should be able to tell you when and how to do this.

Take care of your general health

It's important to look after your own wellbeing. You can do this in the following ways:

Take regular exercise – Start or continue to exercise daily for as long as you can manage comfortably during pregnancy. Experts recommend at least 30 minutes of daily gentle exercise, such as walking or swimming in a warm pool.

Make time to relax – More than at any time during your life, during pregnancy it's essential to get enough rest and make time to recharge your batteries. Whether that means taking a regular relaxing bath or simply finding time to sit and read a book or magazine, make sure that you're looking after yourself.

Reach a healthy BMI – It's important to be a healthy weight before you try to conceive. Body Mass Index (BMI) is a measure of body fat based on height and weight, applying to adult men and women. A healthy BMI is classed as being between 18.5 and 24.9. If you are below this, you're classed as underweight and if you're above it, you're overweight.

Know the risks of being underweight or overweight – Being either underweight or overweight can affect your fertility, although this is not the case with everyone. Being underweight or overweight can also affect your chances of having a healthy pregnancy. Underweight women may struggle to get enough nutrients for themselves and their growing babies. Overweight women are more at risk of developing pregnancy complications such as high blood pressure. We've included guidelines for a healthy diet from page 15 in this chapter.

Tip

Get ready to be in the toilet a lot more often than usual

During the first few months, your womb presses on your bladder, probably making you need to wee more often than usual. In the second trimester, this should ease off. In the third trimester, you'll find yourself needing to wee more frequently again as your baby drops lower in your pelvis, ready for delivery, putting pressure on your bladder again.

Take folic acid and vitamin supplements

Take folic acid – As we've already mentioned, start taking folic acid three months before you try to conceive if possible. You're advised to take 400 micrograms of folic acid (0.4 mg) daily.

WHY? Folic acid helps prevent neural tube defects, which can cause structural problems in your unborn baby's brain and spinal cord. For this reason, you're advised to take folic acid daily until around week 12 of your pregnancy.

Take vitamin D – You're also recommended to take 10 mcg of vitamin D daily throughout your pregnancy and should carry on taking it after your baby is born, if you decide to breastfeed.

WHY? Vitamin D regulates calcium and phosphate in the body – essential for keeping teeth and bones healthy. Taking it during pregnancy will provide your baby with enough vitamin D during their first months. Although vitamin D can be found in eggs, meat and oily fish, it can be difficult to get enough through food alone, which is why a supplement is recommended during pregnancy.

Know which vitamins are safe before and during pregnancy – Some vitamin supplements are not safe during pregnancy. Don't take any high-dose multivitamin supplements, fish liver oil supplements or supplements containing vitamin A as too much vitamin A can damage your baby.

Tip

If you decide to take a nutritional supplement, make sure it's suitable for pregnancy

This should be marked clearly on the packet. If you're not sure, ask your GP, midwife or practice nurse.

Eat a healthy diet

Try to eat a balanced diet – Eating a healthy diet full of vitamins and minerals is important at any stage of life. However, it's vital during pregnancy, when you aren't just supporting yourself – you're growing another person! Around 15 per cent of pregnant Brits are overweight. Yet, healthy eating during pregnancy has been found to prevent diabetes, high blood pressure and even premature birth.

Don't worry if you give in to food cravings – They're one of the most talked-about aspects of pregnancy. Lots of women experience overwhelming food cravings during their pregnancy, whether it's crisps in the first trimester, followed by fresh pineapple in the second trimester – and chocolate cake in the third. A little of what you fancy won't do you any harm but try to maintain a mainly healthy diet for both you and your baby's sake. You may also find yourself attracted to certain scents, depending on which trimester you're in.

Don't fall into the 'eating for two' trap – If you were hoping that pregnancy was the perfect excuse to hit the doughnuts, you're heading for disappointment. Sadly, the old saying 'you're eating for two now!' is very misleading. Under no circumstances should you be eating double your pre-pregnancy calorie intake, even if you're expecting twins or triplets. During pregnancy, your body becomes more efficient by wasting less. Pre-pregnancy, women are advised to consume around 2,000 calories daily. Pregnant women generally need 300 calories more than this – equivalent to one slice of wholegrain toast, half an avocado and around eight almonds.

Choose healthy snacks – Some women find that early pregnancy nausea can only be eased by regular snacks. In this instance, you should choose healthy options (you'll find more details on page 19).

Eat foods containing folic acid – In addition to taking a folic acid supplement, you should try to eat foods rich in folic acid such as:

✓ avocado

✓ raw mushrooms

✓ spinach

✓ broccoli

✓ raspberries

✓ nuts

✓ cooked dried beans

✓ citrus fruits

Eat two portions of fish weekly – Fish is a good source of protein and contains vitamins, minerals and essential omega 3 fatty acids. All adults, including pregnant women, women trying to conceive and breastfeeding mums, should try to eat at least two portions of fish weekly, at least one of which should be oily fish.

Tip

Omega 3 fatty acids for vegetarians and vegans
Vegetarians and vegans can eat flaxseeds and walnuts for essential omega 3 fatty acids, or should consider a specialist, vegetarian supplement – be sure to check that it's safe to take during pregnancy.

Some types of fish should be avoided or limited during pregnancy or pre-conception (see section below). But you don't need to limit or avoid the following fish:

✔ plaice

✔ cod

✔ haddock

✔ skate

✔ hake

✔ flounder

✔ gurnard

✔ coley

Eat five portions of fruit and veg a day – Vegetables and fruit provide vitamins, minerals and fibre, aiding digestion and preventing constipation. They can be:

✔ fresh

✔ canned

✔ juiced

✔ dried

Eat plenty of carbs – Starchy foods provide energy, fibre and vitamins without too many calories. They should be included in every main meal. They include:

- ✓ potatoes
- ✓ sweet potatoes
- ✓ yams
- ✓ bread
- ✓ pasta
- ✓ rice
- ✓ noodles
- ✓ breakfast cereals
- ✓ millet
- ✓ maize
- ✓ oats
- ✓ cornmeal

Choose healthier options of everyday foods – Opt for wholemeal rather than processed, white options. Leave the skins on potatoes because they contain more fibre that way.

Eat two or three portions of dairy foods daily – It's important to include dairy products in your diet because they contain calcium and other nutrients that are vital for your baby's development. Dairy foods include:

- ✓ cheese
- ✓ milk
- ✓ yoghurt and fromage frais

Go low fat – Opt for low-fat versions, such as semi-skimmed or skimmed milk, low-fat yoghurts and reduced fat hard cheese. **There are some cheeses you should avoid when pregnant (see section below).**

Eat protein daily – Foods containing protein include:

✓ meat (but avoid liver)

✓ fish

✓ poultry

✓ eggs

✓ pulses

✓ nuts

✓ beans

Go lean – Opt for lean meat, remove the skin from poultry, and try not to add extra fat or oil when cooking meat. Make sure all meats are cooked thoroughly.

Know which foods to limit

Limit foods high in saturated fats, sugar or both – These are often high in calories and contribute to weight gain and tooth decay. As you are more susceptible to tooth decay during pregnancy, it's important not to overdose on sweets. Fatty, sugary foods also increase the risk of high cholesterol and heart disease. These foods include:

✗ crisps

✗ chocolate

✗ biscuits

✗ pastries

✗ ice cream

✗ cake

✗ puddings

✗ fizzy drinks

✗ oils

✗ butter and margarine

Choose healthy snacks – If you get hungry between meals, opt for healthy snacks such as:

✓ hummus with pitta or vegetable sticks

✓ beans on toast

✓ ready-to-eat fruit such as figs, prunes and apricots

✓ low-fat yoghurt or fromage frais

✓ fruit

✓ sandwiches or pitta bread with ham, tuna, salmon or grated cheese with salad

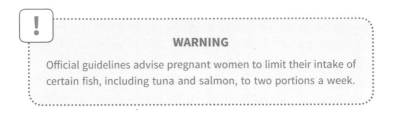

WARNING

Official guidelines advise pregnant women to limit their intake of certain fish, including tuna and salmon, to two portions a week.

Stay up to date with the latest healthy eating advice – We have been careful to ensure that all the information in this book corresponds to the guidance given on the NHS Choices website. For information on the latest official pregnancy guidelines, visit www.nhs.uk.

Try a healthy pregnancy smoothie

This smoothie, devised by nutritional therapist Sally Wisbey, is bursting with nutrition for the healthy development of your baby.

INGREDIENTS

245 g natural yoghurt

1 banana

Handful of mixed berries

1 tsp of ground flaxseeds

1 tsp of chia seeds

1 tbsp of oats

Handful of spinach

- ▶ Natural yoghurt contains high levels of protein – essential for foetal cell growth, brain development and blood production. Prebiotics stimulate good gut bacteria and contribute to a healthy immune system.

- ▶ Oats are high in soluble fibre, which prevent constipation, a common pregnancy symptom. They contain complex carbohydrates to keep energy levels stable and folic acid for prevention of birth defects.

- ▶ Bananas are high in magnesium, which helps prevent pre-eclampsia and poor foetal growth. They also provide potassium, which can prevent headaches and muscle cramps in the mother.

- ▶ Spinach is packed with iron – essential to prevent pregnancy anaemia.

- ▶ Berries are high in antioxidants and flaxseeds are bursting with omega 3 fats. Both are required for the neurological development of your baby and to support baby's brain and eye development.

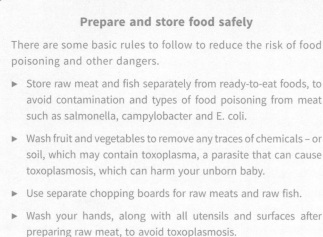

Prepare and store food safely

There are some basic rules to follow to reduce the risk of food poisoning and other dangers.

▶ Store raw meat and fish separately from ready-to-eat foods, to avoid contamination and types of food poisoning from meat such as salmonella, campylobacter and E. coli.

▶ Wash fruit and vegetables to remove any traces of chemicals – or soil, which may contain toxoplasma, a parasite that can cause toxoplasmosis, which can harm your unborn baby.

▶ Use separate chopping boards for raw meats and raw fish.

▶ Wash your hands, along with all utensils and surfaces after preparing raw meat, to avoid toxoplasmosis.

▶ Heat ready meals until they're piping hot all the way through – this is especially important for meals containing poultry.

▶ Ensure eggs, poultry, burgers, sausages and whole cuts of lamb, beef and pork are cooked thoroughly, without any traces of pink.

Know which foods to avoid

Learn which foods should be avoided or limited – There are certain foods which you are advised to avoid when pregnant, or trying to conceive. This is because they could cause food poisoning or contain bacteria, which could harm your unborn baby.

You want to protect your unborn child. However, knowing exactly what you can and can't eat during pregnancy can be tricky, especially when it seems that the official guidelines are constantly chopping and changing.

Check which 'rules' have changed – Until fairly recently, pregnant women in the UK were advised to avoid eating peanuts for fear of causing allergies in their unborn child – if there was a history of any allergy such as asthma, eczema, hay fever or food allergies in their immediate family.

But this advice has now changed. The latest research has shown no clear evidence that eating peanuts during pregnancy can cause your baby to develop a peanut allergy. So if you fancy toast smothered in peanut butter, go ahead (unless you have an allergy yourself, of course).

Check the official guidelines – Visit www.nhs.uk for the latest food advice from NHS Choices.

According to the latest guidelines (as shown on the NHS Choices website at the time of going to press), here's some advice on the foods you should either avoid, limit or treat with caution:

▶ Don't eat unpasteurised cows', goats' or sheep's milk or any food made of them, including soft goats' cheese.

▶ Don't eat soft blue-veined cheeses (such as Danish blue, Gorgonzola and Roquefort) or mould-ripened soft cheeses (such as Brie, Camembert and others with a similar rind, including goats' cheese) uncooked. Cheeses made with mould can contain listeria – a bacteria that cause listeriosis. You can still eat soft, mould-ripened or blue-veined cheeses, if you cook them thoroughly, such as oven-baked Camembert, as the cooking process kills the bacteria. Just make sure they're piping hot throughout.

> ### What is listeriosis?
>
> Although the infection is rare, pregnant women are approximately 20 times more likely than other healthy adults to get listeriosis. In pregnant women, it's typically a mild, flu-like illness. Yet even a mild form during pregnancy can lead to miscarriage, stillbirth or severe illness in a newborn. Pregnant women should also avoid farm animals that are giving birth or have recently given birth. This is to avoid the small risk of infection.
>
> *Note on hard, blue-veined cheeses:* Hard, blue-veined cheeses such as Stilton are less likely to contain listeria than soft, mould-ripened cheeses. The NHS says that Stilton is safe to eat uncooked during pregnancy. However, the risk of listeria contamination cannot be completely ruled out so you may prefer to avoid all blue cheeses unless they're cooked.

▸ Don't eat any type of pâté, including vegetable pâté, which could contain listeria and is eaten without further cooking, once bought.

▸ Don't eat raw or undercooked meat. Cook all meat and poultry until there's no trace of pink or blood.

▸ Treat cold cured meats with caution. The Food Standards Agency (FSA) advises pregnant women to be careful when eating cold cured meats such as pepperoni, salami and Parma ham. Due to being cured and fermented rather than cooked, they may contain toxoplasmosis-causing parasites. If a pack of cured meat is labelled 'ready-to-eat', you can reduce risks by freezing it for four days at home before eating. Freezing kills most parasites.

▶ Don't eat raw or undercooked eggs and any foods containing them, such as home-made mayonnaise. Ensure that eggs are thoroughly cooked until the yolks are set to prevent the risk of salmonella food poisoning.

▶ Don't eat liver or liver products, such as liver sausage or pâté, as they may contain a lot of vitamin A. Too much vitamin A can harm your baby.

▶ For this reason, you also shouldn't take high-dose multivitamin supplements, fish liver oil supplements or supplements containing vitamin A either. Always check with your doctor or midwife before taking any supplements.

▶ The following types of fish should be avoided completely if you're pregnant or trying to conceive. They contain high levels of mercury, which can affect your baby's developing nervous system.

   ✕ shark
   ✕ swordfish
   ✕ marlin

▶ Limit your intake of tuna if you are pregnant or trying to conceive, because it also contains high levels of mercury.

Don't eat more than two tuna steaks a week (each weighing 170 g raw or 140 g cooked) or four medium-sized cans a week (140 g a can when drained).

▶ Limit your intake of oily fish, such as fresh tuna, salmon, mackerel, herring, sardines, pilchards and trout, to two portions a week. This is due to the pollutants they may contain. However, the health benefits of oily fish outweigh the risks if you stay within the recommended amount.

▶ Don't eat more than two portions a week of the following fish either – sea bass, sea bream, crab, halibut, turbot and dogfish – due to the risks of pollutants.

▶ Don't eat raw shellfish as it can cause food poisoning. It's considered safe to eat shellfish providing it's been thoroughly cooked as viruses and bacteria are usually killed through cooking. However, some toxins may not be completely removed by cooking. With this in mind, you may choose to avoid shellfish completely during your pregnancy.

▶ Avoid sushi containing raw shellfish. During pregnancy, you should only eat cooked shellfish (see advice above).

> **!**
>
> **WARNING**
>
> According to the NHS guidelines, it's considered safe to eat sushi and other dishes made with raw fish when you're pregnant. But make sure that it's been frozen first. Occasionally, raw fish such as

salmon contains small parasitic worms, which can make you very ill. However, freezing kills parasites, making it safe. Smoked salmon doesn't need to be frozen before it's used in sushi, because smoking kills any parasites. Salting and pickling also make raw fish safe. Again, however, as with shellfish, you may decide that avoiding all raw fish during pregnancy is easier and more reassuring.

Limit caffeine and herbal teas

Limit your caffeine intake – Many mums-to-be go off tea and coffee, especially during the early stages of pregnancy. If you still fancy a cuppa or soft drink with added caffeine, bear in mind that you're advised to limit caffeine during pregnancy. This is because high levels of caffeine can cause miscarriage or low birth weights in babies. Don't have more than 200 mg of caffeine a day – equivalent to two and a half shots of espresso or two and a half cans of caffeinated energy drink, such as Red Bull.

Limit herbal teas – Although you might consider herbal teas to be a safe option during pregnancy, it's actually best to drink them in moderation. That's because not much is known on how safe herbal and green teas actually are during pregnancy. Also, it's worth remembering that green tea contains caffeine. The FSA (Food Standards Agency) recommends no more than four cups of herbal or green tea a day during pregnancy. If you're unsure about which herbal products, ask your midwife or GP.

Avoid raspberry leaf tea until the last weeks of pregnancy – Raspberry leaf tea is thought to stimulate the uterus and some women credit it with helping them have a shorter labour with more powerful contractions. Whether you choose to believe its effectiveness or not is up to you. But if you do choose to try it, you should avoid drinking it before you are 32 weeks pregnant. If you are at all unsure about drinking raspberry leaf tea, consult your midwife or GP.

Avoid certain herbs – Because rosemary may have uterine stimulant effects, it is best to avoid using it in large quantities such as in tea or as an essential oil for aromatherapy (more on this in the section about beauty treatments later in this chapter). However, small amounts in cooking aren't thought to be dangerous. Other everyday herbs to be avoided drinking in tea during pregnancy include basil, thyme and oregano but, again, they are safe in small amounts for cooking.

Limit alcohol

Know the safe limits – So can you have a glass of Chardonnay during pregnancy… or not? It's a question that befuddles expectant mums. Everyone seems to have an opinion on drinking during pregnancy. It doesn't help that the official guidelines have always seemed unclear. Twenty-five years ago, expectant and breastfeeding women were given stout to boost iron levels. Then mums were advised that it was OK to drink in moderation. But in 2007, the government reviewed the guidelines. Expectant mums are now advised to abstain completely from alcohol for the first three months because of the risk of miscarriage.

WHY? When you drink, alcohol passes through your blood and to your baby, via your placenta. In the first trimester, your baby's liver isn't fully developed. Too much exposure at such a crucial stage can affect their development, lead to birth abnormalities or behavioural problems later on. Research has also found that drinking heavily in early pregnancy can increase the risk of low birth weight and premature birth.

In later months, experts say that, if you can't cut out your alcohol intake completely, you must not drink any more than one or two units once or twice a week (approximately one glass of wine).

Having said that, don't beat yourself up if you drank alcohol before you knew that you were pregnant. You certainly aren't the first and you won't be the last! The chance of one or two incidents is highly unlikely to have a detrimental effect.

Don't be afraid to ask for help – If you have difficulty cutting your alcohol intake, talk to your midwife, doctor or pharmacist. You can also find confidential help and support from local counselling services – contact Drinkline on 0300 1231110.

CHAPTER 2

THE DOs AND DON'Ts FOR GENERAL HEALTH AND LIFESTYLE

PRE-PREGNANCY AND FOR THE WHOLE NINE MONTHS

Taking care of your general health and knowing what is safe during your everyday life is vital for a healthy, enjoyable pregnancy.

Whom you should inform of your pregnancy

While you may not want to shout your pregnancy from the rooftops in the early days, there are some people whom you need to inform in confidence. Your GP needs to know about your pregnancy and, if you have appointments with other medical practitioners during the early stages, you need to tell them too so that they can give you the appropriate advice and care.

Tell your doctor – If you've done a positive pregnancy test at home, your next step should probably be to tell your GP that you're pregnant so that your antenatal care can be arranged and you will be assigned a midwife. Sometimes, GPs like to do another test to ensure that your initial one was accurate but this is not always the case. It's also worth bearing in mind that, as some hospitals operate a self-referral process, you may not need to speak to your GP directly but instead fill in a self-referral form (usually this can be obtained on the hospital's website, if they operate the self-referral system). Then, once you're registered with the maternity unit at the hospital, your GP will also be informed.

Apply for your maternity exemption certificate – Prescriptions and dental care are free during pregnancy until one year after your due date. To get this, you should apply for a maternity exemption certificate. Ask your midwife or GP for form FW8, which they will sign and send off for you. You will then receive an exemption card, which you will be required to show to pharmacists and dentists when you're receiving treatment.

Tell your pharmacist – Your lowered immune system during pregnancy may make you more susceptible to bugs and sniffles. Many over-the-counter medicines aren't safe in pregnancy – or if you're breastfeeding – so always make sure your pharmacist knows that you're expecting.

> **Over-the-counter medicines that are usually safe include:**
>
> ▶ paracetamol – although The Royal College of Midwives advises to always check with your doctor before taking paracetamol during pregnancy
>
> ▶ indigestion relief remedies
>
> ▶ nicotine replacement therapy
>
> For coughs and colds, try safe options such as nasal sprays and honey with hot water and lemon.

Tell your dentist – There are some dental treatments to avoid in pregnancy so make sure that your dentist knows you're expecting. X-rays will probably be delayed until after you've had your baby and your dentist will advise as to whether new or replacement fillings should be fitted afterwards too. It's important to look after your teeth, especially as the pregnancy hormone changes can make your gums more vulnerable to plaque. This can cause your gums to bleed and is known as pregnancy gingivitis, which your dentist can treat.

Tip *Maintaining good oral hygiene during pregnancy*
- ▶ Clean your teeth twice a day for two minutes.
- ▶ Avoid sugary and acidic foods.
- ▶ Avoid mouthwashes containing alcohol.

Don't brush your teeth straight after vomiting – If you're suffering morning sickness, don't brush your teeth immediately after being sick. Your stomach acid will have softened your teeth. Rinse your mouth with plain water instead and wait an hour before brushing.

Look after your skin

Be prepared for skin flare up – Unfortunately, pregnancy hormones can affect your skin in different ways throughout the 40 weeks. This is due to your skin secreting more excess oil. You may notice an outbreak of teenage-like acne or that you're more susceptible to heat rash.

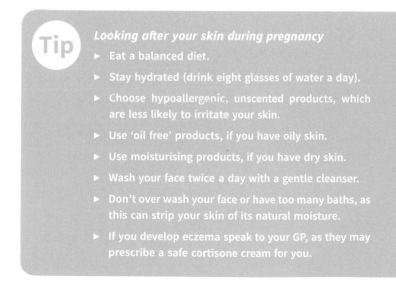

Tip

Looking after your skin during pregnancy

▶ Eat a balanced diet.

▶ Stay hydrated (drink eight glasses of water a day).

▶ Choose hypoallergenic, unscented products, which are less likely to irritate your skin.

▶ Use 'oil free' products, if you have oily skin.

▶ Use moisturising products, if you have dry skin.

▶ Wash your face twice a day with a gentle cleanser.

▶ Don't over wash your face or have too many baths, as this can strip your skin of its natural moisture.

▶ If you develop eczema speak to your GP, as they may prescribe a safe cortisone cream for you.

> ▶ Some women develop skin tags during pregnancy. These usually disappear after delivery or can be easily removed by a dermatologist.

> ▶ If you have heat rash (a pink or red raised rash, which may sting or itch and can appear on any part of skin covered by clothing), try to stay as cool as possible by avoiding tight clothing, wearing natural fibres such as cotton and linen and staying out of the midday heat.

Don't suffer in silence if you have regular, severe headaches – Headaches are quite common in pregnancy. Make sure you're drinking enough water, as dehydration can be a cause. But severe head pain can be a sign of something serious. Check with your GP if you are concerned.

Take regular exercise

Try to stay active – Don't worry; exercise isn't dangerous for your baby! In fact, some research has found that women who are active are less likely to experience problems later on in their pregnancies and labour. The NHS advises mums-to-be to maintain their normal physical activity as long as possible. But don't go over the top. It doesn't have to be strenuous activity, especially if you weren't particularly sporty pre-pregnancy. Walking or swimming is ideal, as are yoga or Pilates, especially classes aimed at pregnant women. Aim for 20 to 30 minutes four or five times a week.

Avoid combat sports – Experts advise against combat sports, such as kickboxing, squash or judo, as there's a chance of being hit.

Don't go scuba-diving – Your baby has no protection against decompression sickness and gas embolism.

Be cautious about sports that have a risk of falls, which could damage your baby – These include horse riding, gymnastics, cycling and skiing. It goes without saying that skydiving is highly inadvisable.

Stop smoking

Giving up smoking is one of the most beneficial things that you can do for your baby – and yourself.

WHY? Every cigarette contains over 4,000 chemicals, along with harmful gases such as carbon monoxide, which harm your unborn baby.

Cigarettes also restrict the oxygen supply to your baby.

BENEFITS TO STOPPING

▶ You're likely to have a healthier pregnancy with fewer complications.

▶ You'll cut the risk of premature birth and stillbirth or having an underweight baby.

▶ You'll reduce the risk of cot death.

▶ Your baby is likely to be healthier in later life, with less chance of suffering conditions such as asthma.

Ask your partner to stop smoking – Second-hand or passive smoke from anyone you live with harms your baby too. If you're trying to give up, it will be easier if your partner is on board too.

> ### Tip
>
> *How to stop smoking*
>
> Call the NHS pregnancy stop smoking advice line on 0300 123 1044.
>
> Ask your midwife or GP about nicotine replacement therapy (NRT). This comes in different forms including patches, gums and nasal sprays and can be used during pregnancy.

Avoid drugs

Know that illegal drugs could seriously jeopardise your and your baby's health – Studies have found that illegal drugs can cause serious complications during pregnancy, including miscarriage and even maternal death. If you're struggling to stop using, your GP may refer you for treatment at your local drug treatment service. Some local drug services accept self-referrals so this is an option if you'd prefer not to speak to your GP. For advice and information, call the Frank drugs helpline on 0300 123 6600.

Learn which beauty treatments are safe in pregnancy

CAN I DYE MY HAIR?

Don't worry, it's generally safe to colour your hair – Some studies have found very high doses of chemicals in hair dye may cause harm to an unborn baby. But most research shows it's safe to colour hair because the amount of chemicals used is miniscule.

You may choose to wait until after the first trimester – The risk of chemicals causing harm is much lower in the later stages.

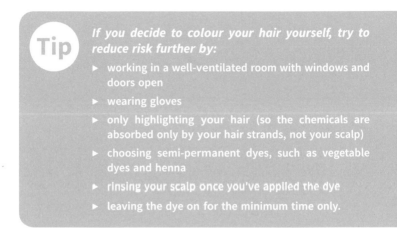

Tip

If you decide to colour your hair yourself, try to reduce risk further by:
- working in a well-ventilated room with windows and doors open
- wearing gloves
- only highlighting your hair (so the chemicals are absorbed only by your hair strands, not your scalp)
- choosing semi-permanent dyes, such as vegetable dyes and henna
- rinsing your scalp once you've applied the dye
- leaving the dye on for the minimum time only.

IS FAKE TAN SAFE DURING PREGNANCY?

Do a patch test if you're using a cream or lotion – Fake tan creams and lotions are generally considered safe to use during any stage of pregnancy. But do a patch test on a small area of skin first to check for allergic reactions.

Avoid spray tans during pregnancy – Experts advise mums-to-be to stop having spray tans. This is because the effects of inhaling the spray are presently unknown.

Don't use tanning pills – Be warned – tanning pills, which are banned in the UK whether you're pregnant or not, contain large quantities of beta-carotene or canthaxanthin. These are commonly used as food colourings and can be toxic to an unborn baby.

ARE BEAUTY TREATMENTS AND SPAS SAFE DURING PREGNANCY?

Treat yourself with a facial or massage – Relaxing with a facial or massage can be lovely during pregnancy. You won't get much chance for treatments once the baby arrives! Some spas and salons even offer specialist mum-to-be packages.

Your second trimester is probably the best time for treatments – Once morning sickness is hopefully behind you but your bump isn't too big for comfort, you'll feel ready for some pampering. If you're feeling sensitive to certain strong smells, you can ask for scentless lotions to be used.

Tell your beautician you're expecting – Do make sure your beautician or therapist is aware that you're pregnant, especially if you're not yet showing so it's not obvious that you're expecting. Some treatments and certain aromatherapy essential oils aren't considered safe to use during pregnancy.

Know which aromatherapy oils should be avoided – It's best to avoid rosemary, nutmeg, basil, jasmine, clary sage, sage, rose and juniper berry as there's a tiny chance that they could cause an adverse effect during pregnancy.

> **!**
>
> **WARNING**
>
> Clary sage – which may trigger contractions – can be found in some toiletries, such as bubble bath and bath oil. Always check the label and avoid anything containing clary sage before you're full term. Some women use clary sage oil from 38 weeks in an attempt to kick-start labour.
>
> *Avoid any lotions containing vitamin A*: It can be harmful to your baby in large quantities. Your therapist will be able to advise you on safe treatments.
>
> *Avoid Jacuzzis, steam rooms and saunas:* If you're visiting a spa, bear in mind that you're advised against using Jacuzzis, steam rooms or saunas during pregnancy because the heat increases your body temperature so dramatically. For the same reason, you shouldn't have very hot baths.

Enjoy nesting safely

Stay safe if you're doing some pre-baby decorating – Most mums-to-be feel the need to 'nest' or get ready for their baby's arrival. It might involve clearing a spare drawer for a selection of tiny babygrows or doing a full-scale redecoration of the house. If you've decided to decorate the nursery yourself, take care. Always ask others to do heavy lifting for you and don't climb up any tall ladders in case you fall. Also, bear in mind that as experts advise new parents to have their baby sleeping in their room at night for the first six months, the decoration of the nursery does not have to be done in a rush during pregnancy.

Avoid painting in the first trimester – It's best to leave the painting to others, especially in the first trimester. Traditional solvent-based paints contain VOCs (volatile organic compounds) – chemical additives that release fumes into the air after you use them. It's not known whether breathing in the chemicals and toxins in paint fumes can have a negative effect on your still developing foetus. But try not to worry if, in your excitement, you've already cracked open the paint tin and done some decorating. It's unlikely that a tiny bit of exposure could do any real harm.

Stay safe when you're painting – In later pregnancy, you should still exercise caution. During pregnancy, try to use low VOC or VOC-free paints, wear a ventilator mask over your face and mouth and cover your skin with clothing. Make sure you finish your decorating well before your due date. Your newborn shouldn't sleep in a freshly painted room, due to the risk of breathing in fumes.

Understand your moods

Be prepared for a rollercoaster of emotions – You're having a baby! You're bound to feel a myriad of emotions ranging from delight, shock, surprise and elation to uncertainty and utter terror. Some women also experience totally unexpected flashes of anger.

Don't be surprised if you feel anxious – You're experiencing a major life change. Having a baby is exciting but it can prompt unexpected anxieties too. Many women report feeling especially unbalanced emotionally during the first trimester. As pregnancy hormones surge through your body, this is perfectly normal so try not to worry too much. Later in pregnancy, you may find that your emotions settle down.

Tip

Ask for help if you need it

Unfortunately, some women develop antenatal depression, a condition that has not been well documented up to now. If you feel down and depressed and your feelings are affecting your everyday life, talk to your midwife or GP in confidence. They will be able to offer help and advise you on the best course of action. If this happens to you, you're not alone.

Talk to your loved ones

If you can, tell your family and friends how you're feeling. Their support – both practical and emotional – will be invaluable.

Learn to deal with unwanted advice

It can sometimes seem that, whatever stage of pregnancy you're at, other people want to offer their pearls of wisdom. Certain advice from people who've been there can be invaluable. However, it can also feel overwhelming to be told what you 'should and shouldn't' be doing, especially if you haven't asked for guidance. It can be a good idea to have a strategy for coping with this. Simply nodding politely and thanking the adviser graciously for their thoughts is often the best way to go, whilst making a mental note not to take their words to heart.

Learn to ignore unhelpful comments – You may find that people feel compelled to comment on the size or shape of your bump. Some may assert that your bump looks 'huge' or 'very small' for your dates, which can send you into a tailspin of worry, especially if this is your first pregnancy and you're feeling self-conscious about your body changes. Rest assured that so long as the medical professionals looking after you are happy with the progress of your pregnancy, you have nothing to worry about. Generally, the best way to deal with people who comment on your shape is to ignore them.

Find support online

Meeting people online isn't solely reserved for lonely hearts wanting dates. There are lots of websites specifically set up to link you with other mums-to-be. Chat forums on websites such as mumsnet have sections where you can 'chat' to other women due to give birth around the same time as you. Comparing notes with people sharing the same experience in real time can be really reassuring. Look on www.mumsnet.com, www.netmums.com and www.babycentre.co.uk.

Understand how pregnancy may affect your relationship

Having a baby, whether it's your first or not, is a huge upheaval and spells change for your relationship.

Make plans together – Planning and looking forward to your new arrival can be an exciting time for both of you. Pregnancy can really bring you even closer and make you feel more loving towards your partner.

Be prepared for hiccups – It's unlikely to be all plain sailing. The change in your situation can also cause difficulties and arguments, especially if one or both of you are feeling nervous about what lies ahead.

Talk to each other – Do try to talk about things with your other half. Be honest and open about your feelings and any fears you may have.

Seek outside help if you need it – If you're in a difficult or abusive relationship, it's important to seek help. The stress of pregnancies can sometimes exacerbate problems. There are organisations that can help, such as Women's Aid (www.womensaid.org.uk) that works to keep women and children safe, or relationship support charity Relate (www.relate.org.uk).

IS IT SAFE TO HAVE SEX?

Don't worry, it's generally considered safe to have sex during pregnancy – Lots of couples find sex during pregnancy enjoyable and satisfying. If you want to, go for it. Your baby won't know anything about it!

Don't be surprised if your sex drive is affected – Hormonal changes during pregnancy may mean that your libido is up and down – and you just don't fancy it. Many mums-to-be report a drop in the first trimester, when they're feeling exhausted and nauseous. But often their sex drive may return with a vengeance in the second trimester!

Know when to avoid it – There are some instances when you should avoid having penetrative sex. These are if you've experienced heavy bleeding recently, or your waters have broken very early during your pregnancy (known as rupture of membranes) and there could be a risk of infection. Check with your midwife if you have any concerns.

Coping alone

It takes two to make a baby. But that doesn't always mean that you face pregnancy and new parenthood as part of a couple. If you're pregnant and don't have a partner, it can be hard to deal with the ups and downs of pregnancy alone.

Find support: It's important to have others around you who can support you, whether they're family or close friends.

Make your own decisions: Remember that this is your pregnancy and your baby. No one else should push you into making any decisions you're not comfortable with.

Meeting other single parents can help: Gingerbread is an organisation that supports one-parent families. It offers advice and information and also has a network of local groups to help you meet other single parents in your position. Call Gingerbread free on 0808 802 0925 or visit www.gingerbread.org.uk.

Be prepared for how pregnancy will affect your working life

If you work full- or part-time, either as an employee or for yourself, you may well find your working day affected by your pregnancy almost from the beginning. You may find yourself struggling to stay awake or away from the toilet, thanks to early pregnancy symptoms such as fatigue and nausea. You may have to consider whether your working conditions are safe or suitable. We will tackle specific points in the following chapters, as you move through your pregnancy.

Know your rights – As a pregnant employee, you have four main rights: paid time off for antenatal care, maternity leave, Statutory Maternity Pay or Maternity Allowance and protection against unfair treatment, discrimination or dismissal.

Know the risks in your workplace – Depending on where you work, you may be exposed to different risks during pregnancy. These may include heavy lifting or carrying, standing or sitting for long periods without adequate breaks, exposure to toxic substances and very long working hours. Remember that it's your employer's responsibility to protect you from these risks. If they can't do this, you should be suspended on full pay until the risks have been resolved or removed.

If you're self-employed, you need to ensure that you look after yourself – If you work for yourself, you have a responsibility to look after your own – and your baby's – wellbeing. That means being clued up on the potential risks of your job during your pregnancy and protecting yourself against them.

Plan for your maternity leave – Legally all new mums have to take a minimum compulsory maternity leave of two weeks – or four weeks if you work in a factory. Some women take up to a year. Maternity leave is an essential time for you to recover from the birth and bond with your newborn. It's a good idea to plan well ahead for this leave – to think about when you'd like to finish work.

Find out about maternity pay or allowance – The thought of taking time off work can be a financial worry. But, if you're currently working, you may be eligible for either:

▶ Statutory Maternity Pay (SMP), paid to you by your employer for up to 39 weeks. You can claim SMP if you've been working for your employer continuously for at least 26 weeks by the end of the fifteenth week before your baby is due. Or if you're earning, before tax, the lower earnings limit for National Insurance contributions which is an average of £109 a week. You have to earn more than this before you start paying National Insurance.

▶ SMP is paid like your wages, with tax and National Insurance deducted. For the first six weeks you'll be paid 90 per cent of your average weekly earnings. For the following 33 weeks, you'll receive the standard rate of £139.58 per week, or 90 per cent of your average weekly earnings, whichever rate is lower.

▶ Some companies pay higher than the Statutory Maternity Pay rates so, if this is the case with your employer, consider yourself very lucky!

▶ Maternity Allowance, a benefit paid by the government for 39 weeks. You may be eligible if you're employed but can't get Statutory Maternity Pay, you're self-employed and pay Class 2 National Insurance for at least 13 of the 66 weeks before your baby is due, or you've recently stopped working. You have to have been employed or self-employed for at least 26 weeks, or earning at least £30 a week over any 13-week period. The amount you get depends on your eligibility.

All the figures quoted above are correct at time of going to press in September 2015 but for the latest information on either Statutory Maternity Pay or Maternity Allowance, speak to your employer, your company's HR department, or go to www.gov.uk.

Ask your partner to look into paternity leave – Your other half may be eligible for two consecutive weeks paid paternity leave, so that they can spend all-important time with you and your newborn. Your partner will need to speak to their employer to find out if they're eligible and how much they'll be paid (some companies pay full pay whereas others only pay basic statutory rate). Your partner will also need to tell their employer your due date so that they can pre-book their paternity leave, if they want to take time off from when you go into labour. For more information go to www.gov.uk.

Know about shared parental leave – Since April 2015, it's been possible for parents to take shared parental leave and claim shared parental pay. So if you want to go back to work before your maternity leave entitlement ends, your partner is legally entitled to take time away from work in order to care for your baby. For more details go to www.gov.uk.

Know about child benefit – All parents are entitled to claim child benefit but if you or your partner have individual incomes of more than £50,000 (correct at time of going to press in September 2015), you may be liable to the high income child benefit tax charge which means that some or all of your benefit payments are taken back. Go to www.gov.uk for details on how to claim child benefit.

Know about tax credits – Child tax credit is a top-up for families, while working tax credit is paid to employees and self-employed people. Both payments are based on your income and the number of hours you work. Child tax credit is paid to the primary carer. Visit www.gov.uk or call the tax credit helpline on 0345 300 3900.

Know your benefits entitlement if you're a single parent – If you're a single parent or on a low income, you may be able to claim other benefits, such as income support, income-based Jobseeker's Allowance (JSA) or Housing Benefit. You can also claim child maintenance, with help from the Child Support Agency (CSA).

If you're not working – You may still be eligible for Maternity Allowance if you've been unemployed during pregnancy but have worked recently (see the section above). Otherwise, you may be eligible for Jobseeker's Allowance, if you're actively looking for work, and other benefits. Visit www.gov.uk for more information.

Travel safely

If you want to travel, do – Whether you're planning a trip away from home for business or pleasure, there's no reason why you can't travel during your pregnancy. A relaxing holiday could be just what you need before your life changes forever!

Choose the best time to go – You might prefer not to go away during the first trimester, if you're suffering from nausea and fatigue. During the first 12 weeks, the risk of miscarriage is higher, wherever you happen to be. By the third trimester, you may prefer to stick close to home as your due date nears. From 28 weeks, many airlines require a doctor's letter to ensure that you're fit to fly. Bear in mind that after 37 weeks (or 34 weeks if you're having twins), your chance of going into labour is much higher. All things considered, the best time to go away is probably between four and six months.

Plan ahead and travel safely – Whatever stage of pregnancy you're at, make sure that you and your baby are covered for any medical eventuality. So it's a good idea to:

✓ Double-check that your travel insurance policy covers you for any complications relating to pregnancy (most do but it's advisable to call up and check or read the small print in your policy).

✓ Apply for a European Health Insurance card (EHIC), which enables you to have state funded treatment in European countries, for free or at a reduced cost. This should not be used instead of health insurance, but alongside it. Find out more at www.ehic.org.uk.

✓ Check whether you need vaccinations for your destination.

✓ Check what medical facilities are close to your accommodation in case you need them.

✓ Take your medical notes with you.

✓ If you're flying long distance, be aware of the increased risk of deep vein thrombosis in pregnant women. Make sure you get up every 30 minutes for a quick walk up and down the cabin.

✓ If you are travelling somewhere hot, remember that you're more susceptible to sunburn during pregnancy – so make sure that you use a high factor suncream, cover up your skin and stay in the shade in the midday sun.

Quotes from experts

DEALING WITH UNWANTED ADVICE

66 Everyone has advice for pregnant women, often unsolicited. Trust your own judgement and seek help from those you can trust, be they health professionals or family and friends. 99

Dr Toni Hazell, GP

ASKING FOR MEDICAL ADVICE

66 Your local community pharmacist is a highly trained healthcare professional who you can easily access without an appointment during pregnancy. Pharmacists know the signs and symptoms of a minor ailment, but they can also recognise something which may require urgent referral for further investigation. 99

Dr Ruth Miller, pharmacist

RELATIONSHIPS

66 Deciding to have a baby is a huge step and commitment. It would be unusual if you and your partner didn't have concerns about how your future life will be. These concerns can become 'niggles' if you don't talk about them. It is important to say what you feel and to listen to what's being said. 99

Denise Knowles, relationship counsellor, Relate

STAYING ACTIVE

66 Staying active during pregnancy is an excellent way of helping stave off or at the very least alleviate many of the pregnancy niggles such as lower back pain, interrupted sleep and swollen ankles in late pregnancy. 99

Dr Joanna Helcké, pregnancy and postnatal fitness expert

DIET

66 Eating for two is a myth. Your food intake at the beginning of your pregnancy should be the same as normal, making sure you're following a healthy diet with lots of fresh fruit and vegetables, good sources of protein and cutting back on foods that are high in refined sugar. 99

Sally Wisbey, nutritional therapist

STOPPING SMOKING

66 Stopping smoking, which results in your baby getting a share of every one of the 4,000 chemicals found in cigarettes, is one of the best gifts you can give your child. Smoking in pregnancy deprives your baby of oxygen, making them more likely to be born underweight; it increases the risk of stillbirth or premature delivery, with all the breathing and feeding problems that brings; it raises the chance of cot death after your baby is born; and it increases your own risk of complications during pregnancy. 99

Dr Sarah Jarvis, clinical consultant, www.patient.info

Quotes from parents and parents-to-be

KNOWING WHAT TO EAT

66 Initially, I was overcautious. But a holiday to France in mid-pregnancy saw me eating cheese, sipping a bit of wine and generally being more relaxed. I think it's each to their own, but I couldn't wait to binge on goats' cheese after my son was born 99

Jo, mum to William, 17 months

MOODS DURING PREGNANCY

66 I usually have very bad PMT. However, I felt emotionally fabulous and level-headed in pregnancy. 99

Katie, mum to Iris, two years, and Arthur, six months

ANNOYING ADVICE

66 Towards the end of my pregnancy, we got sick of people grabbing us and saying 'Your life will never be the same again. Enjoy these last few months of freedom!' Sure, it's all true and sure, we didn't really understand the full magnitude of it at the time. But it was repeated so often by so many people I just wanted to say 'No, really?!? I was just planning to stick the baby in my handbag and go clubbing...' 99

Andreina, mum to Rufus, 18 months

DAD'S VIEWPOINT

" I felt more protective. I was suddenly looking after two people and she was carrying my child. She was protecting our baby so it was my duty to protect them both. **"**

Martin, dad to Archer, 20 months

CHAPTER 3

THE DOs AND DON'Ts FOR THE FIRST TRIMESTER

It's happened, you've hit the jackpot… you're pregnant! Now you're embarking on one of the most exciting journeys of your life. The first trimester – from weeks one to 12 – is a crucial stage of your baby's development. It also means lots of changes for your body, some of which occur before you've even realised that you're expecting.

Learn what happens to your baby – and you

Weeks one to four – Your pregnancy is dated from the first day of your last period. It might sound confusing but this means that, in what's counted as your first two weeks of pregnancy, you aren't actually pregnant.

In those two weeks, you will ovulate – release an egg – which is fertilised. During the third week after the first day of your last period, the fertilised egg moves along the fallopian tube towards the womb.

By the time it's reached your womb, the egg – which began as a single cell – has divided repeatedly to become a mass of over 100 cells called an embryo. It then burrows safely or 'implants' into the lining of your womb. Sometimes, you can actually sense when this is happening because you may feel light cramping in your abdomen. However, lots of women mistake the implantation process for period pains at this early stage.

The embryo stays in your womb lining to grow for the next few weeks. At first, it's nourished by a tiny yolk sac but within a few weeks, the placenta will be fully formed, supplying the baby with a rich blood supply, oxygen and nutrients.

IVF conception

If you've undergone successful IVF treatment, you may be feeling a mixture of emotions – from utter delight to terror that your pregnancy could end in miscarriage. It's understandable that you'll be nervous after the stress of IVF treatment. But once you're pregnant, unless doctors have identified a particular health concern, you should think of yourself as being just the same as any other expectant mum.

By week five – You'll have probably missed your first period – which may be the first sign of your pregnancy and the point at which you take that all-important pregnancy test. At this stage, the embryo is around 2 mm long and its nervous system is already developing, along with a layer of cells called the neural tube, which will eventually form the baby's spinal cord and brain. Simultaneously, the heart is taking shape.

By week six – The embryo is the size of a lentil and covered with a layer of translucent skin. It is curved and has a tail – a bit like a tadpole! It also has tiny swellings called limb buds that will eventually become arms and legs, and dimples on the side of the head, which will become ears.

By week seven – The embryo has grown to 10 mm long and its head is much bigger than the rest of the body because of the rate at which the brain is growing. Cartilage starts to form in the limb buds, which will develop into leg and arm bones.

From eight weeks – The embryo is called a foetus, which means 'offspring'. By this stage, your womb will have stretched to the size of a lemon and you may have experienced 'growing pains' occasionally in the form of light cramping.

By week nine – Your baby's face is forming, with eyes, a mouth, tongue and even taste buds. The heart, brains, lungs and kidneys continue developing and the hands and feet develop ridges, which will eventually become fingers and toes. By now, the baby will have grown to around 22 mm long.

By week 10 – Your baby's heart is fully formed and beating 180 times a minute – up to three times faster than your own heart. Its ears and ear canals are developing, along with an upper lip and two tiny nostrils. By now, its small, jerky movements can be picked up by ultrasound scan.

By week 11 – Your baby is the size of a fig. Its head makes up one third of its length but its body is growing rapidly, and all the bones of its face are formed. The eyelids won't open for a few months yet but it already has fingernails.

By week 12 – The placenta is now fully formed – and so is the foetus, with all its organs, limbs, bones in place, along with its sex organs. All it has to do now is grow! Although the baby is moving around a lot, it will be too early for you to feel anything. So that fluttering sensation you can feel in your belly is probably just wind…

Know what to expect from your antenatal care

Book your antenatal care – As soon as you know you're pregnant, you can contact your GP or midwife so that they can refer you for antenatal care. Your GP surgery or local children's centre can put you in touch with your local midwifery service.

Some hospitals operate a self-referral process, which means that you sign up directly with them, either by phone or online. They will then organise your booking-in appointment, which should take place by the time you're 12 weeks pregnant.

If you have any existing disabilities or health issues speak to your GP or midwife – If you have existing health conditions, which could affect your pregnancy, your GP or obstetrician may have shared responsibility for you during your pregnancy, which means you'll see them for appointments as well as a midwife. Your midwife also needs to know about any health issues so that they can make arrangements for your care during pregnancy and labour.

Know what to expect from your antenatal appointments – If this is your first baby and there aren't any complications with your pregnancy, you will have up to ten antenatal appointments. If you've had a baby before, you will have around seven. Early in your pregnancy, you should be given a schedule of appointments (this may be found within your handheld notes). Don't forget that if you can't make an appointment, you must let the midwife, clinic or hospital know so that you can rebook.

Be prepared for your first appointment – During your first meeting with your GP or midwife, when you tell them that you're pregnant, they will give you information on nutrition, folic acid and vitamin D supplements. Please note that if you self refer to hospital, you may not have this appointment and will be given the information at your booking-in appointment instead.

Know what to expect at your booking-in appointment – This will take place within your first trimester, between your eighth and twelfth weeks of pregnancy. It will take place either at your hospital, a health centre, GP's surgery or at your home. If your partner is available, it's a good idea for them to come with you, for support, because the process can last around two hours.

What will probably happen:

▶ You'll see a midwife and will be offered the chance to book your first ultrasound scan.

▶ You will probably be weighed and will have your blood pressure checked. You will also be asked questions about your general health and your partner's, along with any previous pregnancies or miscarriages or any existing health issues, your family's medical history and any genetic conditions such as cystic fibrosis.

▶ You'll be asked the date of the first day of your last period. It's helpful if you can tell the midwife this so that an approximate due date can be worked out.

▶ You will be given information on the antenatal screening tests that you can have as well as advice on maintaining your general health.

▶ You may also be advised on your options for giving birth – a consultant-led unit, midwife-led unit or a home birth. If you're considered low risk, you can opt for a home birth or to give birth at a midwife-led unit. If your pregnancy has complications and you are considered 'high risk', you may be referred straight to a consultant-led unit. Every expectant mother has the right to request an elective caesarean on the NHS. But it's down to individual consultants to agree to this or not. In some areas, mums-to-be are asked to make this decision fairly early on, whilst others are not pressed for a decision until the third trimester. (There is more information on preparing for a home birth, if you have made that decision, on page 137, Chapter 6.)

▶ You may be given information on breastfeeding, nutrition, exercise and the benefits you may be eligible for.

Be prepared to answer personal questions – The midwife will have to ask you about your lifestyle, your job, how much alcohol you drink along with questions such as whether you intend on breastfeeding. It may be a lot to think about at such an early stage but it's good to start considering the decisions you'll face over the next few months.

Be prepared to give samples – You will probably be asked for both a urine and a blood sample, which will be taken at the time of your booking in. This is so that essential antenatal screening tests can be carried out.

Tell your midwife if you're feeling down or depressed – During your booking-in appointment, your midwife may ask whether you have a history of mental health problems and whether you have experienced antenatal or postnatal depression before. If you're feeling low, don't keep it to yourself. Rest assured you won't be the first – or the last – to feel like this. Tell your midwife, who'll be able to offer help and advice.

Antenatal classes: What's available?

During your booking-in appointment, you'll also be given information on antenatal classes, which take place later in your pregnancy – probably in your third trimester.

NHS classes: All expectant mums are eligible for free classes, sometimes called parentcraft classes, run by NHS midwives. These will take you through the practicalities of labour and giving

---

birth. You may also be able to attend a breastfeeding workshop. As demand is high, you may need to book your place on these classes fairly early in your pregnancy. Your midwife should be able to advise you how and when you should do this.

NCT classes: Another option is to join a local NCT class. The National Childbirth Trust (NCT) runs regional classes focusing on preparing for labour and the process of childbirth, along with advice on breastfeeding. It also offers support and organises social groups for new parents. Classes, which are taught in small groups, aren't cheap (prices vary dependant on location). But many swear by them as the best way to meet local mums all due around the same time. Classes are generally aimed at first-time parents but there are also refresher options for parents who've done it all before. As classes are popular, it may be a good idea to book yourself in as early as possible. To find out more, go to www.nct.org.uk.

Other options: You may prefer to attend other types of classes, such as pregnancy yoga, hypnobirthing (see page 128, Chapter 6) or birthing classes run by individual midwives. Ask your midwife for information on the options in your area.

Know when to worry about bleeding

Don't immediately panic if you experience light bleeding – It can be quite common to have light bleeding or 'spotting' during the first weeks of pregnancy, especially around the time that your period would be due. It's always a good idea to mention it to your midwife if it happens to you, but don't freak out as many women do experience it and go on to have successful pregnancies.

> **!**

Learn about the 12-week scan

Know what to expect from your 12-week scan – You'll be offered an ultrasound scan when you're between eight and 13 weeks pregnant (although some women may have earlier scans if they have suffered previous miscarriages). It's an exciting moment for most mums-to-be the first chance to see a glimpse of your baby! It's sometimes called a dating scan because it gives the sonographer an opportunity to give you an estimated due date, according to the size of your baby.

WHAT IS AN ULTRASOUND SCAN?

▶ Ultrasound scans use waves to build up a picture of your baby.

▶ They are carried out by trained medical staff called sonographers.

▶ Totally harmless to both you and your baby.

▶ Painless – you won't feel a thing (except for, perhaps, the handheld sensor pressing into your tummy) and neither will your baby.

WHAT HAPPENS?

▶ You'll lie on a bed in a dimly lit room so that the sonographer can see good images of your baby on a screen.

► Once you've bared your tummy, the sonographer will smooth ultrasound gel on your tummy. Be warned – it can be cold!

► The sonographer runs a handheld sensor over your tummy. This sends out ultrasound waves and picks them up when they bounce back.

► A black-and-white image of your baby will appear on the screen. This will be your first glimpse of your baby.

Make sure you have a full bladder before your appointment – A full bladder moves your bowel out from your pelvis into your abdomen, helping the sonographer get a clear view of your baby.

Wear something practical – Trousers or a skirt which can be lowered and a top that can be raised to your chest are the best bet for giving the sonographer access to your tummy. Jumpsuits are a bad idea!

Take someone with you – If your partner can come along, that's ideal. It's a special moment for both of you and lovely to share, especially if your baby puts on a good show and waves his or her arms and legs around for you to see! As some scans do show up problems with the baby or pregnancy, it's important to have someone with you for moral support.

Be prepared for it to take a while – You could be in there for 20 to 30 minutes depending on the position of the baby. The sonographer needs to take measurements and make lots of important checks.

If you have requested that your baby is screened for their risk of having Down's syndrome, part of the combined test for Down's syndrome, this will take place during this scan. This is called a nuchal translucency scan (NT) and it looks for increased fluid at the back of your baby's neck, which can be an indication of Down's syndrome. You will receive the results of the screening test within a week or so.

Organise childcare for older children if you can – Many hospitals don't allow children into scanning rooms so it's better if someone else is looking after your older children, if you have any. Check the hospital's policy on children before you go.

Take some spare change to pay for scan pictures – Most hospitals allow you to take away a precious picture of your little one. And no matter how blurred or fuzzy it is, you may well find yourself gazing at that black and white image for weeks and months to come. Most hospitals charge a small fee for photos so make sure you have some cash with you to avoid disappointment.

WHAT HAPPENS IF THE SCREENING TESTS SHOW A PROBLEM?

Try not to worry – Most babies develop normally so it's rare for scans to detect problems. But if the scan does show up anything out of the ordinary, the sonographer may ask for a second opinion from a colleague. You may be offered further tests to determine whether there is a problem and you may be referred to a specialist.

But it's important to be realistic – Sadly one in four pregnancies doesn't make it through to full term. That does mean that it's important to be aware of the risk of having a miscarriage in the early stages of your pregnancy. And, unfortunately, some women receive this sad news at their first scan. That's why, if your partner can't come with you, it's important to take a trusted relative or friend along for moral and practical support.

Coping with bad news – Miscarriage is devastating at any stage. If it happens to you, you may feel a torrent of emotions from intense grief and disbelief to anger. You must give yourself time to recover both physically and emotionally. But the crucial thing to remember is that many women who suffer miscarriage go on to have a healthy baby in the future – and there's no reason why you can't be one of them. For advice and support visit www.miscarriageassociation.org.uk or for more information on miscarriage see page 164, Chapter 7.

Health: be prepared for how your body may be affected by the 'worst' trimester

It's unlikely you'll see any sign of a bump during the first weeks of your pregnancy. However, you're likely to gain some weight and see thickening around your waist as the trimester progresses. Some women do start to show in the first trimester, especially if it's not their first pregnancy.

For some women, missed periods are the only signs that they're pregnant. But for others, the symptoms are more dramatic. You may experience a heightened sense of smell, which will have you noticing cigarette smoke, aftershave or body odour at 50 paces.

Some of the early signs of pregnancy can be debilitating. Although pregnancy isn't an illness, it can make you feel physically awful at times, especially in the first few weeks.

In fact, some people refer to the first trimester as the 'worst trimester' because of the effects on your overall wellbeing.

Learn strategies to deal with tiredness, sickness and other unpleasant symptoms

Yes, it's normal to feel this tired – From around week seven, you may experience the sort of utter, all-consuming exhaustion which sees you dropping off on the sofa as soon as you get in from work. You may even start craving daytime shut eye. This sudden need to nap is caused by the high levels of the hormone progesterone in your system.

Don't fight the desire to rest if you don't have to – You need all the sleep you can get in the first trimester.

Ironically, although you will probably be more tired than usual, you may also suffer disturbed sleep, which is again caused by heightened levels of progesterone. You may also find yourself snoring in your sleep – something that may affect your partner more than you!

Sore, swollen boobs may be making it impossible to get comfortable in bed, especially if you're used to sleeping on your front.

> **Tip**
>
> *Get used to sleeping on your left side as you sleep, even in early pregnancy*
>
> Lying in this position improves the flow of nutrients and blood to your womb – and your baby. It also helps your kidneys expel waste.

TOILET BREAKS

Don't be embarrassed about needing the toilet – You may find yourself rushing to the toilet, needing to wee more frequently, because your growing womb is putting more pressure on your bladder.

Accept that wind and bloating are part of pregnancy too – Some women also experience bloating and wind due to the hormone progesterone that your body produces early in pregnancy. Again, don't be embarrassed about this. It's just one of the many slightly undignified – but essential – indications of your body changing to accommodate your growing baby.

NAUSEA AND SICKNESS

Be prepared for morning sickness – Most people have heard of 'morning' sickness but the name is misleading because pregnancy sickness is rarely confined to the first part of the day. You may be one of the lucky 20 per cent of pregnant women who don't experience it at all. But around half of all pregnant women experience vomiting, and more than 80 per cent of women feel nauseous in the first few weeks.

There's even a chance that you may suffer all-day nausea or sickness. It can be hard to deal with when you're trying to carry on as normal or keep your pregnancy under wraps in the early stages.

Tip

Dealing with nausea and sickness

► It's important not to stop eating, as many women find their nausea worsens when they're hungry.

► Eating small amounts, frequently, rather than large meals, may help.

► Sip fluids, such as water, little and often rather than at once.

► Avoid cold, tangy or sweet drinks.

► High-carb, low-fat savoury foods (bread, rice and pasta) are preferable to spicy or sweet foods.

► You may find it easier to eat cold rather than hot food as it won't have such a strong smell.

► Give yourself time to get up in the morning rather than rushing.

► If possible, eat a plain biscuit or some dry toast before you get out of bed.

► Explain how you're feeling to those around you and ask for support.

► If strong smells spark nausea, it may be easier for someone else to cook.

> ▶ Some evidence suggests that ginger supplements may reduce symptoms. As ginger products are unlicensed in the UK, always buy from somewhere reputable and check with a pharmacist.
>
> ▶ Some women find that ginger biscuits or ginger ale help.
>
> ▶ Wearing an acupressure band on your wrist may reduce nausea symptoms.
>
> ▶ Tiredness and stress can worsen nausea so get plenty of rest and relaxation.

When will it end?

For most women, nausea and sickness tend to ease by 14 weeks but for one in ten women, symptoms unfortunately last beyond 20 weeks. Pregnancy sickness can grind you down – don't be afraid to ask for support and help if you're struggling.

Know about extreme morning sickness

Recognise the signs of extreme morning sickness – Some women are diagnosed with an extreme form of morning sickness and nausea, called hyperemesis gravidarum. It can cause sufferers to vomit up to 50 times a day, making it impossible to keep fluids and food down.

It's thought to affect around one in every 100 women. Kate Middleton famously suffered with hyperemesis gravidarum during both her pregnancies.

If you're concerned that you're suffering from it, seek help – Don't try to suffer in silence and soldier on. It's a debilitating condition that can lead to serious complications including malnourishment, dehydration, ketosis, serious weight loss and low blood pressure.

If you're drinking less than 500 ml of fluid a day and have lost weight during the first weeks of your pregnancy, you must get help from your GP or midwife.

Sufferers may be prescribed anti-sickness medication and, if vomiting cannot be controlled, you may be admitted to hospital for treatment including intravenous drugs given directly through a drip, to rehydrate you.

Thankfully, although severe morning sickness is awful to experience, it's unlikely to harm your baby.

Eat healthily and safely

Eat a balanced diet – It's important to try to eat healthily during your first trimester, with a diet rich in vitamins and minerals. But the reality is that if you're feeling nauseous, you may only be able to stomach certain foods, some of which may not be classed as the healthiest options. Just do your best to have as balanced a diet as possible. (For tips on eating a balanced diet, look at the guidelines from page 15, Chapter 1.)

Eat safely – For information on the current guidelines for foods that are safe during pregnancy – and those that should be avoided – see pages 18–31, Chapter 1.

Know the risks of alcohol, smoking and illegal drugs in early pregnancy

Be clued up about the official advice on alcohol – In the first trimester, you may feel too queasy to even sniff a bottle of wine, let alone drink from it. But is it safe to have a drink or not? As discussed in Chapter 1, expectant mums are now advised to abstain completely from alcohol for the first three months because of the risk of miscarriage. That's because, in the first trimester, your baby's liver isn't fully developed. Exposure at such a crucial stage can lead to birth abnormalities or behavioural problems later on. Research has also found that drinking in early pregnancy can increase the risk of low birth weight and premature birth.

> ### Don't be afraid to ask for help
>
> If you have difficulty cutting your alcohol intake, talk to your midwife, doctor or pharmacist. You can also find confidential help and support from local counselling services – contact Drinkline on 0300 1231110.

Give up smoking for your baby's sake – As already discussed, giving up smoking is one of the most beneficial things that you do for your baby. For more details go to pages 37–38, Chapter 2.

Know that taking illegal drugs could seriously jeopardise your and your baby's health – As discussed in Chapter 2, taking illegal drugs during any stage of your pregnancy can cause devastating results. For more details see page 38, Chapter 2.

Limit your caffeine intake

Know the risks of too much caffeine – You're advised to limit the caffeine you consume during pregnancy. For more information on the safe limits, see page 29, Chapter 1.

Get fitted for a bigger bra

Look after your changing breasts – If, like many women, you find your breasts and nipples feel suddenly enlarged and tender to touch during the first trimester, you may need to get fitted for a bigger bra. Underwired bras can feel restrictive and some experts think that the wire may press against your developing milk duct system. For comfort's sake, you may prefer to wear a soft cup style. Many high street stores, such as Marks & Spencer and Mothercare, offer free measuring services for maternity and nursing bras and will offer advice on the best style for your shape. As your breasts continue to grow during your pregnancy (and will grow considerably more once your baby is here and your milk comes in!) you may need to getting fitted regularly during your pregnancy. For this reason, it's more economical to buy cheaper styles. You may also find that stretchy crop top styles accommodate your changing breasts for longer.

Exercise safely and sensibly

Try to stay active but listen to your body – The NHS advises mums-to-be to maintain their normal physical activity as long as possible. Research has found that mums who stay active are less likely to experience complications during pregnancy and may find it easier to cope with labour. But it's important to be sensible.

Don't force yourself to exercise if you feel ill – If you're suffering pregnancy fatigue or sickness in your first few weeks of pregnancy, the last thing you'll feel like doing is pulling on your trainers and going for a jog. Use your common sense and listen to your body. If you need to rest, then do. For information on the best types of exercise – and which ones to avoid – go to pages 36–37, Chapter 2.

Understand your changing moods

Accept that your emotions may be unpredictable – In the first trimester, lots of mums-to-be feel that their emotions change rapidly due to raging hormones. And, don't forget, you're experiencing a major life change. Having a baby is exciting but it can cause you to feel more anxious than usual.

If you're happy one moment but weeping the next, try not to worry – It's completely normal for your emotions to be unsettled at this stage. They should balance out as your pregnancy progresses.

Ask for help if you need it – If your feelings and anxieties are affecting your everyday life, talk to your midwife, who will be able to offer help and advice.

Be prepared for how early pregnancy may affect your relationship

Be prepared for changes in your relationship – You've made a baby together! The excitement should hopefully bring you closer to your partner. But don't be surprised if it also causes you both to feel unsettled about the future, especially in the first trimester when the reality of pregnancy is all so new. It may even spark arguments as you both adjust.

Be open with each other about your feelings – Do your best to be a partnership now and it'll be easier to stick together once the tricky business of parenthood begins.

Accept that you might not feel like sex – When it comes to the physical side of things, you may not feel much like being touchy-feely with your partner or having sex in your first trimester. Your sex drive will change throughout pregnancy and sex will probably be the last thing on your mind if you're suffering from nausea, sickness or fatigue. If you feel like this, do talk to your partner about it.

Don't worry, sex is safe – If you do want to have sex in early pregnancy, it's perfectly safe. Your partner's penis can't penetrate beyond your cervix – and the baby won't know a thing!

Work out which position is right for you and your changing body – You may find that some positions are difficult at this stage. If your breasts are sore, sex with your partner on top can be uncomfortable. It may be better to lie on your sides, facing each other or with your partner behind.

Get help if you are in an abusive relationship – Sadly, difficult relationships sometimes become even more so during pregnancy. If your partner is abusive or violent towards you, get help from an organisation such as Women's Aid at www.womensaid.org.uk.

Find support right from the start if you're on your own

Don't try to cope on your own – If you're pregnant and don't have a partner, it's important to have support from those around you right from the beginning.

Ask for support – It can be hard attending your first medical appointments alone so try to get someone you trust to accompany you. But remember that this is your baby and it's your pregnancy. If you feel that a friend or relative is trying to take over, try to tell them politely that any decisions are yours to make.

Know how early pregnancy may affect your working life

Coping with work during the first trimester can be hard, especially if you're suffering early pregnancy sickness and tiredness.

Try to use your breaks to rest – Don't rush around, running errands, during your breaks. You need to rest and retain your strength when you can.

Keep healthy snacks at your desk – If you need regular snacks to keep nausea at bay, make sure you have a healthy selection within easy reach during the working day (for tips on healthy snacks, go to page 21, Chapter 1).

If you're employed

Know about workstation assessments – Your workstation should be checked at regular intervals during your pregnancy, from the first trimester, to ensure that you are not at risk.

Make sure you're safe – If there's a recognised safety risk associated with your job, such as heavy lifting or working with lead, X-rays or chemicals, it may be illegal for you to continue working in these conditions. Legally, your employer must offer you suitable alternative work on the same terms and conditions as your original job.

Decide whether to tell a colleague about your pregnancy in confidence – If you're finding your daily routine difficult, it could be a good idea to tell someone – a colleague or your line manager – in confidence so that you have their support if needed. Your employer may even agree to allow your working different hours, to avoid a difficult commute in rush hour.

If you're self-employed

Start looking into Maternity Allowance – If you're registered as self-employed, you are probably eligible to receive Maternity Allowance, a benefit paid to pregnant women by the government. You may also be eligible if you haven't been working for your employer long enough to receive Statutory Maternity Pay or if you are an employee and your average wage is less than £112 a month (correct at time of going to press in July 2015). Visit www.gov.uk for more information on Maternity Allowance.

Be a kind boss to yourself – While being your own boss can be fantastic, it can also mean that you only have yourself to rely on, which can be hard in the first few months if you're feeling tired and nauseous. You also have a responsibility to look after yourself. Make sure that your workstation is suitable. Ensure that you're not risking your or your baby's health. Most of all, listen to your body and don't push yourself too hard.

Travel safely

Be prepared if you're going on holiday – You might prefer not to go away during your first trimester, especially if you're suffering nausea and fatigue. Flying in pregnancy does not pose a risk to your baby but bear in mind that, wherever you are, the first 12 weeks hold the most risk for miscarriage. However, a holiday could also do you the power of good in the early stages. So if you decide to go away, you should take a few steps to ensure that you and your baby are safe (for tips on travelling safely, go to pages 51–52, Chapter 2).

Quotes from experts

MEDICINES

66 Many medicines are unsafe during pregnancy. It does depend on the trimester – many drugs are particularly lethal during the first trimester when the foetus is developing rapidly. It's essential to check with a healthcare professional prior to taking any medicine. 99

Dr Ruth Miller, pharmacist

MORNING SICKNESS

66 Be sure to eat small healthy portions and not let yourself get hungry. Do not be tempted to eat high sugar foods. Instead eat protein snacks. Sip water with ginger grated into it. Be reassured that sickness indicates a healthy pregnancy and should pass when the second trimester is reached. 99

Virginia Howes, midwife

SEX

66 Losing your libido in early pregnancy isn't uncommon. You'll have concerns about the viability of the pregnancy, the safety of your unborn baby and how you feel about yourself too. Maintaining intimacy sensually rather than sexually will go some way to ensuring distance doesn't grow between you and your partner at this time. Talking and sharing worries will help develop understanding and trust at this time of transition. 99

Denise Knowles, relationship counsellor, Relate

TALKING TO YOUR GP ABOUT ANY CONCERNS

66 Pregnancy is an exciting time, though it can be an anxious one too. GPs are always happy to answer questions about health in pregnancy, though for minor symptoms the advice of a friend or relative who has been pregnant herself may be just as useful! 99

Dr Toni Hazell, GP

Quotes from parents and parents-to-be

NOTICING THE EARLY SIGNS

66 My boobs ached, my period was overdue and I just felt... different. A bit of Googling and I thought it wise to do a test and – *voilà*! – there was the line. I was five weeks. 99

Jo, mum to William, 17 months

66 I nearly burst into tears because my husband didn't bring me a cup of tea when he said he would. I wanted to scream at him, but I told myself not to overreact, and decided to buy a pregnancy test the following day. Early on, I had really tender breasts. I had to suppress yelps whenever my daughter cuddled me! 99

Grace, 19 weeks pregnant and mum to Evie, two years

66 I had really vivid dreams, which made me guess that I was pregnant because I never normally remember my dreams. I was

constantly trying to remember whether something had happened in real life or not. **"**

Jennifer, 16 weeks pregnant

COPING WITH FIRST TRIMESTER FATIGUE

" In the early weeks, I'd have to take naps on my desk, then lie down the moment I got home from work and not move until I went to bed at 8 p.m. I couldn't help my husband cook, clean, walk the dogs, do the shopping or anything. **"**

Becca, 13 weeks pregnant

COPING WITH MORNING SICKNESS

" I had severe nausea from weeks six to 13. It was worst in late afternoon and the middle of the night, and I had crackers by the bed for middle of the night nausea. **"**

Katie, mum to Iris, two years, and Arthur, six months

COPING WITH HYPEREMESIS GRAVIDARUM

" From week five, I was being sick several times a day, couldn't swallow my saliva or keep fluids down. I couldn't picture coping with nine months feeling so ill. Eventually, a midwife diagnosed me with HG, and took me to A&E to be rehydrated on a drip. After being prescribed a strong anti-sickness medicine to prevent me vomiting, I finally felt brighter and more in control. **"**

Grace, 19 weeks pregnant and mum to Evie, two years

KNOWING WHAT WAS SAFE TO EAT

66 The night I found out that I was pregnant, I went out and ordered a medium rare burger, with soft cheese and mayonnaise. Afterwards, I realised what I'd done! I did get used to the 'rules', but not until after I'd checked what foods I could eat about 20 times. 99

Gemma, mum to Amelie, six months

HOW DID THE PREGNANCY AFFECT YOUR RELATIONSHIP?

66 For the first nine weeks, it was our little secret, which brought us closer. We loved sharing that exciting but terrifying time together. 99

Gemma, mum to Amelie, six months

MOOD SWINGS DURING THE FIRST TRIMESTER

66 I was very grumpy and had huge mood swings. We were moving house at the time. My husband wouldn't let me talk on the phone to the estate agent in case I shouted at him. 99

Linda, mum to Harry, 16 months

DEVELOPING A SUPER SENSITIVE SENSE OF SMELL

66 I found smells really hard to deal with in the beginning. My husband's shower gel and aftershave made me feel sick, so he was banished to the spare room. 99

Georgina, 39 weeks pregnant and mum to Arabella, two years

SEEING BABY ON SCREEN AT 12-WEEK SCAN

66 I felt total and utter relief to see my baby. I couldn't believe it. It's a miracle, I truly believe that. One of the most magical experiences. 99

Clare, mum to Isabelle, two years

SEX IN THE FIRST TRIMESTER

66 It's not so much a loss of libido – more that I've felt so deathly, sex is the last thing on my mind! 99

Lynsey, 13 weeks pregnant

COPING WITH WORK

66 I told my boss when I was five weeks pregnant. I work in a potentially hazardous environment so needed to make sure that I was safe. 99

Jennifer, 17 weeks pregnant

CHAPTER 4

THE DOs AND DON'Ts FOR THE SECOND TRIMESTER

You've made it through the first trimester and have now entered the second trimester. For many women, this stage is the most enjoyable part of pregnancy. You may start to feel more like your old self again, with the early symptoms of pregnancy fading. There are also lots of exciting changes happening to your body. This is the stage where you'll really start to see and feel definite signs of your pregnancy. As your baby's growth accelerates, you should see the appearance of that all-important bump. You'll also have some important check-ups and an ultrasound scan, which may be able to tell you of your baby's sex. All in all, a very exciting trimester indeed.

Learn what's happening to your baby

By week 13 – Your baby is now the size of a peapod and weighs around 25 g. Excitingly, its sex has now been determined. The nub between its legs will be forming into a clitoris or penis. So is it a boy or a girl? You impatient types have a while longer to wait. You generally can't find out the sex of your baby at an ultrasound yet. Most NHS hospitals offer to disclose the sex at the 20-week anomaly scan, whilst some private clinics offer 'gender' scans from 15 weeks.

By week 14 – Your baby is now around 85 mm from head to bottom. Its kidneys are starting to work, which means that it can swallow tiny amounts of amniotic fluid that pass through its body and back out into the amniotic fluid as urine.

By week 15 – Although your baby's eyes are still fused shut, they're becoming sensitive to light. Its ears are also starting to hear, which means it can hear muted sounds from outside your body, including your voice.

By week 16 – Your baby is the size of an avocado and weighs around 100 g. The muscles in its limbs and face are developing, meaning that it can make a fist and form facial expressions, although It has no control over them.

Between 17 and 19 weeks – Your baby is growing quickly and will weigh around 150 g at this stage. It also looks more like a human (than an alien!), with eyebrows and eyelashes and a mouth that moves. Incredibly, it already has its own unique fingerprint. Your baby is moving around and may respond to loud noises such as music or your voice. You may feel these movements for the first time. Some mums say it feels like butterflies fluttering in their stomach.

By 20 weeks – You're halfway through your pregnancy! Your baby is the size of a banana. It's now covered in a thick layer of 'vernix', a white, waxy substance that protects its skin *in utero*. Many babies are born with traces of vernix on their bodies, which can be easily wiped off.

Between 21 and 23 weeks – Your baby will weigh around 350 g. It will also grow a covering of very soft, fine hair known as lanugo. It's thought to keep the baby at the right temperature and usually disappears before birth. Although its lungs aren't working properly and it's getting all its oxygen through the placenta, your baby is practising breathing movements to prepare for the day it's born. It may also be adopting a pattern of waking and sleeping, although not in sync with yours. So you may experience lots of fluttering movements just as you're nodding off at night!

By 24 weeks – Your baby now weighs around 600 g. This is the point at which your baby would have a chance of survival if it were to be born, although it would be very premature. Before 24 weeks, most babies would not live because their vital organs and lungs just aren't developed enough. Sadly, babies born this early do have an increased chance of disabilities and long-term health issues. They will require many months of specialist care in a neonatal unit before being well enough to go home – and many need ongoing treatment.

For help and advice on premature births, go to www.bliss.org.uk.

Learn what's happening to you

Get ready to experience the long awaited 'bloom' of pregnancy – Lots of people talk about the second trimester as being the most enjoyable. Hopefully, you'll start feeling more like your old self again. Most women leave any morning sickness and nausea behind by week 16.

But if you're not yet blooming, you're not alone

Unfortunately, some unlucky mums-to-be do find that nausea, sickness and fatigue continue beyond 20 weeks. If this is your experience, it can be hard to stay buoyant, especially if you know other pregnant women who are back to their normal selves. You're certainly not the only one to have a difficult time. Be kind to yourself and get plenty of rest. Make sure you have good practical and emotional support around you. If you're struggling with prolonged sickness, do seek help from your midwife or GP.

Make the most of it if you feel better – If you do find that you have more energy again, keep active although don't tire yourself out – by doing regular exercise. You may fancy joining a specific pregnancy related class at this stage, such as pregnancy yoga or aqua aerobics. Not just an ideal way to get fit, going to classes are a great way to meet other expectant mums in your area. (For more advice on the best exercise during pregnancy, see page 36, Chapter 2.)

Watch out for your baby's first movements

Your baby is moving around a lot and you may feel its movements for the first time around 17 to 20 weeks. Some women describe it as feeling like 'butterflies fluttering' or a whooshing or rolling sensation.

But try not to worry if you can't feel anything at first – The movements are initially so subtle that you might mistake it for indigestion so don't worry if you think you haven't felt anything yet. If you have an anterior placenta placement – which means that your placenta is positioned at the front of your bump, cushioning movements, you may not feel movement until later. Rest assured that by the time you reach the third trimester, you'll be getting kicked and elbowed from within at regular intervals!

Don't be surprised if you feel movements in the middle of the night – If, like many women, you find that your baby is most active at night or at the crack of dawn, you may feel those all-important movements just when you're trying to sleep! That's because your constant movement during the day tends to lull your baby to sleep inside the comfort of your womb. Although it is lovely to feel your baby's flutterings, it can be frustrating when you're exhausted and trying to get some rest. Try to get some rest during the day if you can too.

But do speak to your midwife if you haven't felt anything by 24 weeks – If you aren't feeling movements by this stage, mention it to your midwife who will be able to offer you guidance.

Prepare for your body's changing shape

Buying maternity clothes, trying to avoid stretch marks, noticing that your breasts may be leaking milk and waiting for your bump to 'pop' – there's a lot to keep you busy in your second trimester!

Go shopping for some maternity clothes – Developing a small bump is the first visible sign that you're pregnant. For many women, it's the most exciting part, along with feeling their baby's movements for the first time.

Look at bump bands – One good stop-gap option can be a belly bump, a piece of stretchy fabric which fits around your tummy and covers the waistband of trousers and skirts, concealing the fact that you can't do them up to the top! They're available from maternity-wear sections of high street stores and some supermarkets. They cost around £10 for a multipack.

Don't worry if your bump doesn't 'pop' until later on – First-time mums generally show later as their stomach muscles are stronger. Depending on whether it's your first or not, you may notice your stomach start to 'pop' from around 14 weeks but others don't notice anything much until 17 weeks or even later. Your belly can suddenly grow very quickly and you may notice changes with each passing day. It's good to have comfortable, looser clothes ready to wear, as your normal clothes become too tight.

Moisturise your bump daily to reduce the chance of getting stretch marks – Your skin has a lot of stretching to do. Stretch marks may appear as silvery lines from around 22 weeks. To reduce the chance of stretch marks, it's a good idea to use a moisturising lotion on your growing bump from fairly early on. Massaging your belly morning and night can be a lovely bonding routine too. There are specialist oils and lotions aimed at pregnant women. However, many mums-to-be find that basic cocoa butter lotion, available at most pharmacists and supermarkets, does the trick. Just make sure that any oil or lotion you choose is safe to use during pregnancy. Check with a pharmacist if you're unsure.

Don't be alarmed if you develop a dark vertical line down your abdomen – This is normal skin pigmentation known as the 'linea nigra'. It's just a sign of your body changing to accommodate your growing baby. The linea nigra usually disappears shortly after giving birth.

You may not need to visit the toilet quite so much – During the first few months, your womb will have been pressing on your bladder, probably making you need to wee more often than usual. In the second trimester, this should ease off.

> ### Talk to your doctor if you feel pain when you wee
>
> Unfortunately urinary infections can strike during pregnancy. Tell your GP if you notice any pain when you wee, as you'll need treatment to reduce the risk of developing a kidney infection.

Don't be surprised if your breasts start leaking milk – As your body prepares for your newborn, your boobs may get in on the action a little early, from around 21 weeks. You can wear breast pads (disposable or washable options are available from pharmacists or supermarkets) to avoid leakage on your clothes.

Make the most of your blossoming body – You may notice that your skin feels clearer and your hair feels thicker during your second trimester, due to a reduction in normal hair loss. You may also notice that your leg hair and armpit hair growth slows down. During this stage, many mums-to-be say they feel full of energy and *joie de vivre*. Enjoy it!

Know how your sex life may be affected during pregnancy

Revel in the return of your libido – Lots of women find their sex drive makes a reappearance during the second trimester, after going AWOL during the first months. This is thought to be due to pregnancy hormones or increased blood flow to the pelvic area.

But don't worry if you don't feel like sex – Lots of women still find their libido is missing in action. This is nothing to worry about. Just make sure you talk to your partner and tell him how you're feeling. Working together as a partnership is vital during pregnancy and beyond.

Know when sex should be avoided – Your midwife or doctor will probably advise you to avoid sex if you've had any heavy bleeding in pregnancy or if your waters have broken early (known as rupture of membranes) as it can increase the risk of infection.

Be prepared for appointments, including your 16-week midwife check-up and 20-week anomaly scan

16-week midwife check-up

Know what to expect from your 16-week appointment – You should have an appointment to see your doctor or midwife at 16 weeks. This may take place at your GP's surgery, at hospital, at a separate clinic or at your home.

Be prepared to give a urine sample and have your blood pressure measured – You'll be asked to give a urine sample, which will be tested for protein. Although small amounts of protein in your urine is normal, larger amounts can be a sign that you're developing pre-eclampsia, a potentially serious condition which can cause dangerously high blood pressure in pregnant women (for more information on pre-eclampsia see page 162, Chapter 7). For the same reason, your blood pressure will be measured and recorded at every midwife appointment.

Be prepared to discuss the results of any screening tests – Your midwife may want to go through the results of tests with you.

Consider taking an iron supplement if you're at risk from anaemia – Almost a quarter of women in the UK are diagnosed with iron-deficiency anaemia during pregnancy and you're most at risk if you eat a vegetarian or vegan diet or are still in your teens. During pregnancy, you need 14.8 mg of iron every day to keep oxygen pumping to your vital organs through your blood – and to keep your baby healthy. If a blood test finds that your iron levels are lacking, your midwife may diagnose iron supplements to boost them.

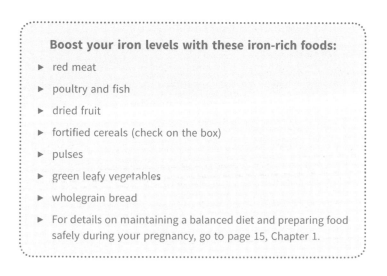

Boost your iron levels with these iron-rich foods:

► red meat

► poultry and fish

► dried fruit

► fortified cereals (check on the box)

► pulses

► green leafy vegetables

► wholegrain bread

► For details on maintaining a balanced diet and preparing food safely during your pregnancy, go to page 15, Chapter 1.

20-week scan

Know what to expect from your 20-week scan – Between 18 and 21 weeks pregnant, you'll be given an appointment for your second, mid-pregnancy ultrasound scan. As is the case with your first scan, this is not obligatory. But, for many parents-to-be, this is a momentous day. That's because it's the point at which you may be able to find out the sex of your baby. However, that's not the actual reason for this scan. It's known as an anomaly scan and its purpose is to check for any potential development issues or major physical defects, although be aware that it's not possible for the sonographer to detect every possible problem. Like the 12-week scan, this scan should take around 30 minutes.

Arrange childcare for any older children – Many hospitals don't allow children into ultrasound scanning rooms. So it's best to have prearranged childcare if you have any older kids.

Take someone with you for support – It's likely that your partner will want to be at this scan, especially if you are going to find out the sex of your baby. But if that's not possible, do try to have someone with you for support.

WHAT HAPPENS?

This detailed scan will proceed just as your 12-week scan did. The sonographer will put ultrasound gel on your tummy and rub a sensor over your skin, in order to pick up a 2D picture of your baby, which will appear in black and white on a screen. You'll be in a dimly lit room so that the sonographer can get a good look at the screen.

The sonographer will look in detail at your baby's heart, brain, bones, spinal cord, face, abdomen and kidneys, and take a number of measurements. It will also look for rare but serious birth defects.

Try not to worry – Most scans are happy occasions. The chances are that your baby is perfectly healthy. But in the unfortunate event that the scan detects a problem, your sonographer is likely to call in a colleague for a second opinion, before referring you to see a specialist so that you can receive further information and support.

Tell the sonographer if you want to know the sex of your baby – Make sure you speak up at the beginning of the scan if you want an answer to that all-important question: boy or girl? If you do want to know, the sonographer should be able to tell you by looking at that all-important area between your baby's legs. If you don't want to know, they'll keep shtum.

Remember that nothing is guaranteed – Nothing is 100 per cent certain at this stage. There have been some parents who've been told their baby is a girl, only to get a surprise at the birth – and vice versa! So it's a good idea not to rush out and buy a mountain of pink or blue items emblazoned with your child's chosen name just yet. Also, if your baby is being coy and is in an awkward position, there's a chance that the sonographer won't be able to detect the sex for you.

Some hospitals won't disclose the sex – Finding out the sex is not offered as part of the national screening programme so your sonographer is not obliged to tell you. Some hospitals have a blanket policy of not confirming the sex. It's a good idea to find out before your visit to avoid disappointment.

Know the official advice about alcohol during the second trimester (and beyond)

Know the official advice about alcohol consumption – As detailed in the previous chapter, the government advises mums-to-be to abstain from drinking alcohol throughout pregnancy, especially during the first trimester, when it can increase the risk of miscarriage.

Be aware of the risks – In the later stages of pregnancy, drinking can affect how your baby grows and also increases the risk of premature birth and low birth weight. If you do choose to drink during your second trimester, you shouldn't drink more than one or two units once or twice a week.

WHY STICK TO THE GUIDELINES?

Drinking heavily (more than six units a day) can cause your baby to develop foetal alcohol syndrome (FAS), a serious condition that can cause your baby to be born with lifelong facial abnormalities, restricted growth and learning and behavioural problems.

Working out alcohol units

One UK unit is 10 ml of pure alcohol, which is equal to:

▶ half a pint of beer, lager or cider at 3.5 per cent alcohol by volume (ABV: you can find this information on the label).

▶ a single measure (25 ml) of spirit, such as whisky, gin, rum or vodka, at 40 per cent ABV.

▶ half a standard (175 ml) glass of wine at 11.5 per cent ABV.

If you have difficulty cutting your alcohol intake, talk to your midwife, doctor or pharmacist. You can also find confidential help and support from local counselling services – contact Drinkline on 0300 1231110.

Exercise safely

You may not feel like going for a jog or a bike ride as your baby gets bigger and your bump grows. You may also develop backache.

Try these handy exercises from pregnancy and postnatal fitness expert, Dr Joanna Helcké.

ROUTINE 1: Resistance band seated pull downs

One of the best things to do during pregnancy is keep the postural muscles strong as this will help stave off back pain.

1. Sit tall on a birthing ball or chair with good posture: shoulders back and down, neck long, chest lifted and abdominals pulled gently inwards.

2. Hold the resistance band above your head with arms wide, chest open and knuckles pointing upwards so that the wrists are aligned.

3. Now lower your elbows to shoulder height, whilst keeping the hands directly above your elbows and squeezing your shoulder blades together.

4. The elbows will be more or less at a 90-degree angle and the chest is wide open.

5. Lift and lower in a slow and controlled manner for ten repetitions. Rest and then have another go if you wish.

ROUTINE 2: Superman

This is a fantastic all-round exercise and is ideal for both during and after pregnancy. It helps with posture and keeps the deepest layer of abdominals toned. NB If you are suffering from pelvic girdle pain (SPD) then you must only do the arm movements.

1. Set yourself up in a box position, on all fours with your hands underneath your shoulders and your knees under your hips.

2. Extend one arm in front of you but keep the fingers lightly touching the floor. Make sure that you are drawing your abdominals inwards so as to avoid arching your lower back.

3. Keep your back level when you lift your arm. Breathe and hold the position.

4. Swap over and lift the other arm. Think about lengthening through your back and arm.

5. Now repeat this process with each leg: lift up your leg without arching your lower back, keeping your toes lightly on the floor; do not tilt your pelvis upwards; breathe.

6. Now put these two moves together and lift opposite arm and leg, following the same movement.

Pelvic floor exercises

Strengthen your pelvic floor: Your pelvic floor muscles, the layers of muscles that stretch from the pubic bone to the backbone, have to cope with a lot of strain during pregnancy and childbirth. It's not surprising that lots of women experience 'leakage' in their knickers when they sneeze or cough. This is known as stress incontinence and if it happens to you, try not to be embarrassed because it's very common. You can wear protective pads to catch leakage but strengthening your muscles can help you reduce or avoid it.

How to do pelvic floor (Kegel) exercises:

- ▶ Make sure your breathing is relaxed.
- ▶ You can do the exercises sitting or standing.
- ▶ Clench your buttocks to close your anus as if you're preventing a bowel movement.
- ▶ Draw in your vagina and your urethra as if to stop urine flow.
- ▶ You should feel a lifting/squeezing sensation inside your vagina.
- ▶ Do this exercise quickly, tightening and releasing the muscles immediately.
- ▶ Then do it slowly, holding the contractions for as long as you can before you relax.
- ▶ Try to do three sets of eight squeezes every day.
- ▶ Also practise tightening up the pelvic floor muscles before and during coughing and sneezing.

Know how your relationship may be affected as your pregnancy progresses

Talk to your partner about your changing body – As your bump develops and your body changes, you and your partner may revel in the exciting changes. But if you're feeling self-conscious, talk to them and be honest so that they can reassure you.

Plan for the coming months – It's a good idea to talk to your partner about how you envisage the rest of the pregnancy going. Would you like them to attend antenatal classes? Do you want them there at the birth (and do they want to be there? If not, why not?)

Don't be afraid to ask your partner for practical and emotional support – It's important to work as a team during pregnancy. Tell your other half when you're tired and emotional and when you need them to help out or give you a confidence boost or pep talk – or some much-needed practical support.

Ask your partner how they feel – Parenthood isn't just going to change your life forever – it will change your partner's too! Ask them how they feel and encourage them to talk about any concerns.

If you are in an abusive relationship, ask for help – Sadly, the stresses of pregnancy can sometimes highlight or even trigger issues. If you are in an abusive relationship, get help now. Contact Refuge for advice at www.refuge.org.uk.

Decide on your birthing partner (whether you have a partner or not)

Make sure you have support at the birth – You'll need support during the birth and if your baby's father is not around, or your partner does not want to attend, it's a good idea to think of someone who can step in as birthing partner. Most hospitals allow you to have two birthing partners. Choose someone you can trust, who wants to be there and can give you practical and emotional support when you need it most. It's a good idea to plan for the birth now so that you can ask your chosen birthing partner if they are willing to be there – and to give them an opportunity to prepare for such a big responsibility. Some women choose to enlist a doula as a primary or additional birthing partner. A doula is a woman – often medically trained – who gives support and help during pregnancy and labour. If you want to hire a doula, you must do this privately. They cannot take the place of the midwife assigned to deliver your baby.

Plan for your maternity leave (whether you're employed or self-employed)

If you're employed

Start thinking about maternity leave – Now you're in your second trimester, you need to decide when you'd like to take your maternity leave. It may seem early but, legally, you must have informed your employer of your intent to take maternity leave at least 15 weeks before your due date. If you're not taking Statutory Maternity Leave, you must take two weeks off after the birth – or four weeks if you work in a factory. This is known as compulsory maternity leave and it's the law.

Tell your employer you're pregnant – You may not have wanted to share your news in the first trimester, before your 12-week scan. But, as we've already mentioned, all employees are legally obliged to tell their employer about their pregnancy at least 15 weeks before the baby is due. Bear in mind that you can't take time off for antenatal appointments before you've told your boss about your pregnancy.

Inform them in writing – Check with your HR department whether they'd prefer an email or letter. You need to tell your boss your due date and the date you'd like to start your Statutory Maternity Leave and Pay.

Collect your MATB1 form – You probably won't have heard of this form before now but it's very, very important and you can't get maternity pay without it. Your midwife should give you the form at your antenatal appointment which takes place after your 20-week scan. But you may need to give your midwife a nudge and ask for it yourself. Your midwife or GP should sign the form and you will also need to sign it.

Give the form to your employer before you're 25 weeks pregnant – To avoid your maternity leave and pay arrangements being delayed, you must give the signed form to your employer or HR department before you're 25 weeks pregnant (15 weeks before your due date). However, some mums-to-be may find that their midwife or GP won't sign their form before they're 25 weeks pregnant – or that they don't actually see their midwife until they're around 24 or 25 weeks pregnant. In this case, it's a good idea to speak to your employer or HR department to let them know that you will give them your form as soon as you get it – so that your maternity leave and pay can still be arranged accordingly.

Know what to do if you can't get Statutory Maternity Pay – Some employed women aren't eligible for maternity pay. But they should be able to claim Maternity Allowance instead – see below for more details. Be aware that you will need an SMP1 form to do this.

If you're self-employed

Start thinking about applying for your Maternity Allowance – If you're your own boss, you're not eligible for Statutory Maternity Pay. However, you can claim Maternity Allowance, a benefit paid to all self-employed pregnant women by the government. You can claim your Maternity Allowance once you've been pregnant for 26 weeks so it's a good idea to get clued up about what you need to do in order to prepare to claim.

Fill in your MA1 claim form – The MA1 claim form is your ticket to your Maternity Allowance. You won't get anything without it. You can find it on www.gov.uk: either print it off and fill it in by hand or fill it in online, print it off and then post it to the address on the form. As mentioned above, you can claim from 26 weeks and payments can start 11 weeks before your baby is due. If you want to claim as soon as possible, it's a good idea to have everything sorted before you hit your third trimester.

Know what paperwork you need to claim – Along with your MA1 form, you'll need to provide: proof of income (payslips, Certificate of Small Earnings Exemption), proof of the baby's due date (letter from GP or midwife or MATB1 form). If you are claiming because you're not eligible for Statutory Maternity Pay from your employer, you also need an SMP1 form.

Know when to expect an answer – You should hear back about your claim within 14 working days. Providing you are eligible and your claim has been accepted, you will be sent another form to confirm your entitlement. You will be asked to confirm your last day of employment before you go on maternity leave.

If you're unemployed – We've provided information on the help and benefits you may be eligible to receive on pages 48–51, Chapter 2. It's a good idea to start looking into this now so you're fully prepared when your baby arrives. For more information visit www.gov.uk.

If you're a single parent – You will be eligible for financial help in the form of benefits and you may also be able to receive child maintenance payments, with help from the Child Support Agency (CSA). For more information, go to www.gov.uk.

Travel safely

Be prepared if you're going on holiday – With the tiresome symptoms of the first months behind you, you may decide that the second trimester is the best time to get away for a break. Flying during pregnancy does not pose a risk to your baby. However, remember that long-haul flights do heighten the risk of deep vein thrombosis in pregnancy. So make sure you get up every 30 minutes to stretch or have a quick walk up and down the cabin. If you're going on a long car journey, make sure you get plenty of breaks in order to stretch your legs. You should always wear your seat belt and make sure it's fitted correctly around your bump.

How to fit your seat belt correctly

1. Strap the lap section of the belt across your thighs and under your bump, not across it (as the pressure across your belly could cause damage).

2. The diagonal shoulder section should go across your collarbone, between your breasts.

3. Fasten it so that it sits above your bump not over it.

For tips on staying safe abroad during pregnancy go to pages 51–52, Chapter 2.

Quotes from experts

TACKLING SNIFFLES DURING PREGNANCY

66 Pregnancy is a difficult time to develop a cold, sore throat or high temperature. First, rest and ensure good fluid intake. The only safe medicine to take in this situation is paracetamol. Check with a pharmacist that no decongestants or antihistamines are included. If an antibiotic is deemed necessary, your GP can safely prescribe a suitable one. 99

Dr Ruth Miller, pharmacist

ADVICE FOR PARTNERS OF EXPECTANT MUMS AS THEIR BODIES CHANGE

66 Your partner may need to feel that she is attractive full stop; this is not just about her body changing. Some women misread reassurance as requests for sex. Confidence is about so much more. Simply being there and supporting her, listening to her self-doubts and giving her time will all contribute to a progressive improvement. 99

Denise Knowles, relationship counsellor, Relate

HEALTHY SNACK OPTIONS

66 Dark chocolate has been proven to have several health benefits. Just eat in small quantities and aim for over 70 per cent cocoa. Medjool dates taste delicious spread with almond or peanut butter. Natural plain yoghurt topped with berries, chopped nuts and

cinnamon is high in protein and antioxidants required for bone and brain development. For an alternative to crisps, chop a sweet potato into wedges, drizzle with olive oil, pink Himalayan salt and paprika and oven roast for 40 minutes. A small handful of olives and chunks of cheddar cheese is high in calcium, which is required for bone development. **"**

Sally Wisbey, nutritional therapist

Quotes from parents and parents-to-be

ON ENJOYING THE SECOND TRIMESTER

" After a pretty grim first trimester, I'm revelling in the second trimester. I have bags of energy, my hair feels thick and my skin is clear. I can also eat normally again, which is a huge relief. **"**

Lisa, 19 weeks pregnant

" I definitely experienced the glow of the second trimester. My skin and hair were lovely. I had an impressive cleavage too! **"**

Katie, mum to Iris, two years, and Arthur, six months

FOOD CRAVINGS

" I couldn't get enough of strawberries, fresh pineapple and kiwi fruit. Weirdly, I couldn't look at porridge, scrambled eggs or mashed potato. **"**

Jo, mum to William, 17 months

❝ I had to have a daily fix of pancakes covered in freshly squeezed orange juice. **❞**

Susie, mum to Bridget, 13 months

DAD-TO-BE'S POINT OF VIEW ON SEEING THEIR PARTNER'S BODY CHANGE

❝ I love seeing her body change. It never ceases to amaze me what happens within the body during pregnancy. **❞**

Will, partner of Hilary, 18 weeks pregnant

CHAPTER 5

THE DOs AND DON'Ts FOR THE THIRD TRIMESTER

The finish line is in sight. You've reached the third trimester – the final straight. Your baby is growing bigger with each day and so is your bump. By now, there will be no disguising that you're pregnant!

Learn what's happening to your baby

Between 25 and 27 weeks – By this stage, your baby's lungs, brain and digestive system are fully formed. They'll spend the rest of your pregnancy developing, ready for his or her birth. Your baby's heart rate has slowed to around 140 beats a minute. It's still much faster than your own heart rate. Your baby responds to sound and touch and moves around quite frequently and vigorously. You'll get used to being kicked at regular intervals! You will even feel it when your baby gets hiccups – which can happen quite often. Around this time, your baby's eyelids will open for the first time too.

By 28 weeks – Your baby is perfectly formed and will weigh around 1 kg. They just need to grow and put on weight, as more fat forms under their skin.

Know about your baby's movements

It's important to be clued up about how often your baby is moving in later pregnancy but it can be confusing to know how much is 'normal'.

Tip

How often should your baby be moving as you near your due date?

According to charity Count the Kicks, it's a misconception that you should be feeling ten kicks over a set period of two hours. All babies are different. Your baby's movements may vary from four kicks to over 100 in the space of two hours. The most important thing is to be aware of your own baby's pattern of movement and stay aware in the last few weeks. If you notice your baby's movements have changed considerably, or stopped or slowed down, contact your midwife straight away.

For more information go to www.countthekicks.org.uk.

Learn what's happening to you, including increased antenatal appointments and experiencing Braxton Hicks

During your third trimester, you will have increasing antenatal appointments, during which your midwife or doctor will:

▶ measure the distance from the top of your womb to your pubic bone to check your baby's growth

▶ feel your tummy to check the baby's position

▶ check your urine and blood pressure (to check that you're not developing pre-eclampsia – explained on page 162, Chapter 7)

▶ listen to your baby's heartbeat if you want them to (tell the midwife if you'd prefer not to hear it).

All these measurements, including your bump growth, your blood pressure and your baby's heartbeat, will be recorded in your notes. You'll be offered a hospital ultrasound scan if there are any queries over your baby's growth or development.

Try not to worry – Remember that, if a midwife refers you for an extra scan to check your baby's growth, or further checks to determine their position, it's not necessarily anything to worry about. Be reassured that health professionals always err on the side of caution in order to give the best possible care. Usually, further investigations will find that your baby is growing perfectly normally. Even if it's found that your baby is in an unusual position – such as in the breech position (when the baby is positioned with its feet and bottom facing down, rather than being head first) – this is something that can be worked around and prepared for when it comes to giving birth.

You'll also be given information on writing your birth plan, preparing for labour, birth and the first few weeks with your baby, along with explaining NHS screening tests for newborns.

Be aware of your baby's movements in the third trimester – Towards the end of your pregnancy, it's important to keep track of your baby's movements. It's a myth that babies don't move as much during the last few weeks.

Be prepared for Braxton Hicks contractions – As your body prepares for giving birth, you may experience a few 'false alarms' in the form of Braxton Hicks. This is when the muscles of your womb tighten. If you place your hands on your belly, you may be able to feel your uterus momentarily become hard. They will probably only last around 30 seconds and shouldn't cause you any pain. They may occur a few times a day and are just a sign of your cervix getting shorter and stretchy, ready to dilate for birth. But don't worry if you don't notice them at all.

Tip

Know the difference between Braxton Hicks and labour contractions:

Braxton Hicks:
- ✓ are usually irregular and infrequent
- ✓ last less than a minute
- ✓ don't increase in intensity

Labour contractions:
- ✓ are regular and frequent
- ✓ are more painful
- ✓ are noticeably longer

Try perineal massage – The perineum is the area of tissue between the vagina and anus. You may not have been particularly aware of it pre-pregnancy but now it's time to become acquainted! Massaging this area regularly in the six weeks leading up to giving birth can prevent tearing during labour.

WHY DO IT?

During birth, the perineal tissues must stretch a great deal to allow your baby's head to be born. Without effective stretching, it can tear. Sometimes, to avoid tearing or during an assisted delivery (e.g. forceps or ventouse), an episiotomy may be required – this is when the tissue is cut in order to make it easier for the baby to be born.

HOW TO DO IT

Many women prefer to do this sort of massage alone in the privacy of their bedroom or bathroom, although some may ask their partner to do it for them.

You'll need

▸ Natural massage oil – such as sweet almond oil, olive oil or a water-based lubricant such as KY Jelly. Don't use petroleum-based products for perineal massage.

▸ A large mirror if you're doing the massage yourself.

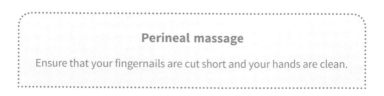

Perineal massage

Ensure that your fingernails are cut short and your hands are clean.

Sitting with your legs apart, place a few drops of your chosen oil onto your fingers and thumbs and then massage the outside of the perineum in a circular motion.

Insert both your thumbs into your vagina (about half a thumb length in) and stretch the perineum until you feel a slight sting. When you feel this, you should maintain the stretch for a minute.

Use your thumbs to massage the oil in a circular motion down to the base of your vagina and also up the sides in a 'u' motion.

Do this for five to ten minutes daily.

Enjoy the nesting stage – Many women report an uncontrollable desire to declutter and redecorate their living space, especially during the third trimester. This commonly felt need to prepare for the arrival of your little one, even though baby really won't care that the carpets are brand new, is generally known as 'nesting'. If you're in the throes of it, do remember to stay safe – or better still, get someone else (your partner, for example) to do it!

Look after yourself if you're doing DIY – As we discussed in Chapter 1 you should leave heavy lifting to others and avoid climbing up tall ladders, in case you fall. If you're doing some painting, exercise caution by following these rules to keep yourself and your baby safe:

✔ Choose low or zero VOC (volatile organic compounds) paint.

✔ Leave the windows open while you paint and afterwards so that any fumes dissipate.

✔ Wear gloves, long trousers and a long-sleeved top to protect your skin.

✔ Wear a ventilation mask with a filter.

✘ Don't eat or drink in the room you're painting.

✘ Don't sleep in a newly painted room.

✘ Don't let your newborn sleep in a freshly painted room either, so make sure that you do it well in advance of your due date – at least a month before.

Eat healthily and deal with cravings and indigestion

Continue to eat a balanced diet in your third trimester – There's no getting around the fact that you will gain weight during pregnancy. You're making a baby after all. Most mums-to-be can expect to gain between 8 kg (17 lbs) and 14 kg (30 lbs), most of it in the second half of the pregnancy, as the body puts down fat in order to produce breast milk. The most important thing to remember is that you need to stick to a balanced diet throughout pregnancy (for more on what you should eat see pages 15–21, Chapter 1).

Stick to a safe diet – Although you're nearing the end of your pregnancy, you should still try to follow the guidelines for 'safe' foods and safe food preparation (see page 24, Chapter 1). The same guidelines apply to the consumption of alcohol (details on pages 30–31, Chapter 1).

Know how to deal with heartburn and indigestion – As your bump grows, you may find that you feel full very quickly. You may also find that certain foods cause heartburn or indigestion. Talk to your GP if you're really suffering and they may prescribe an antacid, such as Gaviscon, which can also be purchased over the counter at pharmacies.

Tip

Indigestion and heartburn relief

If you're suffering from heartburn and indigestion, follow these top tips from nutritional therapist Sally Wisbey:

- ▶ Avoid eating late at night and eat little and often.
- ▶ Chew your food well and avoid fatty, greasy or sugary foods, as these are acidic.
- ▶ Mix one teaspoon of apple cider vinegar with water and sip before each meal to help digestion.
- ▶ Fennel tea after a meal can aid digestion but avoid tea and coffee as these can be acidic.

Don't be surprised if you start craving sweet treats – Lots of women report cravings for cake and chocolates during the later stages of pregnancy so don't worry if you're dreaming of sugary treats. Some experts think that this could just be your body stocking up on energy before the birth. There's no harm in the odd cake or chocolate. But try not to overindulge too much and choose healthy snacks, such as bananas or porridge, which release energy more slowly.

Be prepared for unpleasant late pregnancy side effects

Be prepared for some less than pleasant side effects in late pregnancy – Unfortunately, as your bump reaches maximum capacity and you near your due date, you may experience some of the less pleasant effects of pregnancy. In Chapter 7, we discuss pregnancy complications – but if you can't wait until then, here are some less-than-glamorous complaints you may come across in your third trimester.

Varicose veins – These are veins which have become swollen and twisted and may be blue or purple in appearance. They usually occur on the legs. They develop when small valves inside the veins stop working, causing blood to flow backwards and collect. They're common – one in three people suffer from them – and pregnancy can increase the chance of them developing, especially in later pregnancy. This is due to the weight of the uterus creating pressure on your veins. You can lower your risk by avoiding sitting or standing still for long periods, taking regular breaks and raising your legs when resting. Exercise improves circulation, which also helps. Varicose veins usually disappear after pregnancy but some women do need treatment for them in the future.

Swollen feet and ankles (also known as oedema) – This is quite common and, in fact, around half of women experience swelling in this area, especially in later pregnancy. It can also affect your hands – you may notice rings getting tight on your fingers. The swelling is caused by water retention and may get more noticeable as the day goes on. Hot weather can also make it worse. To ease symptoms, put your feet up as much as possible and don't stand for long periods of time. You may find support tights helpful. The swelling should subside as soon as – or soon after – you have given birth.

> **!**
>
> **WARNING**
>
> If your face, hands or feet swell up very suddenly and severely, call your doctor or midwife. Sudden swelling could be a sign of pre-eclampsia, a serious condition, which we discuss on page 162, Chapter 7.

Piles (or haemorrhoids) – These are swollen veins around the anus, which may feel like small lumps and may bleed slightly. They may itch or feel sore, especially when you go to the toilet. Mums-to-be are especially prone to piles because the pregnancy hormones, which make your veins relax, can cause them to form. Constipation can also cause piles. You can ease piles by eating a diet high in fibre and staying hydrated. Regular exercise can also help. Your GP may prescribe safe medicines or pain-relief creams. Thankfully, most piles disappear within weeks of giving birth.

Be clued up about late pregnancy vaccinations

Consider having the flu vaccination – The NHS offers a free flu vaccination to all pregnant women. It's usually available between September and February each year – the traditional flu season.

WHY SHOULD YOU CONSIDER THE VACCINATION?

Pregnant women are advised to have the jab because they're more likely to develop complications such as bronchitis and sepsis (severe blood infection). If you catch flu, the effects on your developing baby can be devastating. Speak to your midwife or doctor to find out more about the vaccination. Remember that even if you had a vaccination the previous year, you will need to be re-vaccinated to avoid new strains of flu.

Have a whooping cough vaccination – All pregnant women are advised to have the whooping cough vaccination when they are around 28 to 32 weeks pregnant, although it can be given up until 38 weeks.

WHY IS IT SO IMPORTANT?

Sadly, whooping cough can be fatal in newborns and cases have been on the rise in recent years. Although you may have had the vaccination as a child, its effectiveness will probably have worn off by now. By being vaccinated during late pregnancy, your immunity will be passed to your baby to protect them before their first vaccination when they are two months old. Speak to your midwife or GP about having the vaccination, if they have not offered it to you.

Know about group B strep

Be clued up about group B strep (GBS) – It's not unusual to carry group B strep – either in your normal gut flora or in your vagina. It does not pose any health risks to the carrier. It can, however, be dangerous – even fatal – if your baby contracts the infection during labour, although only a very small percentage of babies develop the infection. If you're found to be a carrier, you should be offered intravenous antibiotics from the start of your labour to protect your baby. Unlike other countries, there are no standard tests for group B strep in later pregnancy in the UK, although it can sometimes be detected during urine tests in earlier pregnancy checks. Private tests are also available for a small fee. Ask your midwife or GP for advice or for more information visit www.gbss.org.uk.

Know what to expect from sex in late pregnancy

Be prepared for sex to set off Braxton Hicks contractions – Sex during later pregnancy is perfectly safe, unless you've been advised against it by your midwife or doctor. But be aware that having an orgasm can set off Braxton Hicks contractions. This is perfectly normal so don't worry. Some people say that, if you're overdue and are desperate to start labour, having sex can be an effective method!

Arrange your maternity leave and pay

You must have told your employer about your pregnancy by now – Remember that, as an employee, you're legally obliged to tell your employer about your pregnancy and your intent to take maternity leave, along with handing over your MATB1 form, at least 15 weeks before your baby is due. If there is any delay with handing over your MATB1 form, it may disrupt your maternity leave and pay arrangements.

If you're self-employed

Apply for your Maternity Allowance – As mentioned in the previous chapter, if you work for yourself, you can't claim Statutory Maternity Pay. However, you're eligible for Maternity Allowance, a benefit paid to all self-employed pregnant women by the government. You can claim your Maternity Allowance once you've been pregnant for 26 weeks and it can start 11 weeks before your baby is due.

Fill in your MA1 claim form   If you haven't already done so, you need to get your hands on your MA1 claim form, which is how you apply for Maternity Allowance. You can find it on www.gov.uk: either print it off and fill it in by hand or fill it in online, print it off and then post it to the address on the form.

Know what paperwork you'll need in order to claim – Along with your MA1 form, you'll need to provide: proof of income (payslips, Certificate of Small Earnings Exemption), proof of the baby's due date (letter from GP or midwife or MATB1 form). If you are claiming because you're not eligible for Statutory Maternity Pay from your employer, you also need an SMP1 form.

Know when to expect an answer – You should hear back about your claim within 14 working days. Providing you are eligible and your claim has been accepted, you will be sent another form to confirm your entitlement. You will be asked to confirm your last day of employment before you go on maternity leave.

Call for advice if you're confused – If you're totally and utterly flummoxed by all this (and no one would blame you if you were), call Jobcentre Plus (Monday to Friday, 8 a.m. to 6 p.m.) on 0800 055 6688.

Whether you're employed or self-employed

Be clued up about keeping-in-touch days – Whether you're employed or self-employed, it's good to know that you're allowed ten 'keeping in touch' days during your 39 weeks of paid leave. This means that you can work for ten days without your maternity pay or allowance being docked. If you work more than this during your paid leave, it will affect what you are eligible for.

Travel safely

Be prepared if you're going on holiday – There's no reason why you can't travel in your third trimester. However, many airlines – and some ferry companies – require a doctor's letter stating that you are 'fit to fly' from 28 weeks. From 37 weeks, you have a heightened chance of going into labour (34 weeks if you're carrying twins) so it's important that you are aware of the potential outcomes and are covered for any eventuality. For tips on safe travel during pregnancy, including checking your travel insurance policy and always carrying your notes, go to page 52, Chapter 2.

Quotes from experts

GET TO KNOW YOUR BABY'S KICKS

" Every baby is different so it is important to get to know their individual pattern of movement. The number of movements tends to increase until 32 weeks when they will plateau as you near your due date. Movements should not reduce as you near your due date and the baby should continue to move up until and during labour. If you're concerned that your baby is moving less or moving much more than usual, seek medical help and get your baby checked. "

Elizabeth Hutton, CEO of Count the Kicks, pregnancy and stillbirth awareness charity

STAYING AWARE OF YOUR BABY'S MOVEMENTS

" A well, healthy baby will move every day. Therefore the opposite is also true. It is vital a woman is aware of her baby's movements so that any irregularity can be checked out. "

Virginia Howes, midwife

STAYING FIT IN LATER PREGNANCY

" Water supports the bump and gives a wonderful feeling of lightness. It can be a great relief to get into water in later pregnancy. With the support of the water, injuries are far less likely to occur, the bump is supported and any feelings of heaviness disappear giving mums-to-be much needed respite in those last weeks. "

Dr Joanna Helcké, pregnancy and postnatal fitness expert

PREPARING YOUR RELATIONSHIP FOR NEW PARENTHOOD

66 Talking, listening and maintaining an interest in one another are essential. Developing day-to-day intimacies like holding hands, snuggling in together and kissing really go some way to couples staying connected. Understanding that tiredness and new responsibilities can impact heavily at this time is useful. Not taking things personally also helps! 99

Denise Knowles, relationship counsellor, Relate

Quotes from parents and parents-to-be

NESTING

66 The final weeks of my pregnancy saw me crouched on the floor, despite my massive bump, painting skirting boards with non-toxic paint. I'd decided that my precious newborn couldn't be brought home to tatty skirting boards. It was nesting gone mad. 99

Liz, mum to Martha, three years

COPING WITH A BIG BUMP

66 Getting in and out of bed was hard during the last weeks of my first pregnancy. I had to roll out! I couldn't clean the shower as my bump was in the way and shaving my legs was very tricky. 99

Kelly, 18 weeks pregnant, and mum to Ben, ten months

CHAPTER 6
THE DOs AND DON'Ts FOR PREPARING FOR GIVING BIRTH

As your due date approaches, you may be feeling a mix of excitement, uncertainty and trepidation. The idea of giving birth can be frightening but rest assured that generations of women have been through it safely and have gone on to have more babies too! The best way to approach your birth is by being as prepared as possible. Here we talk about the ways in which you – and your partner – can do this.

Attend antenatal classes

Antenatal classes can be invaluable – You have the option to attend free NHS classes or private ones, run by organisations such as NCT. These classes aren't compulsory but, if this is your first pregnancy, it's a good idea to attend them. You'll learn tips about preparing for birth, coping with labour as well as learning about those all-important first weeks and months with your newborn, whether you've chosen to go to NHS classes or another option (read about the options on pages 63–64, Chapter 3). Although you'll probably have had to book your place on these classes fairly early in your pregnancy, you will attend them during your third trimester. Attending classes, with or without your partner, is also a great way of meeting other local parents-to-be.

Consider learning hypnobirthing techniques – Increasing numbers of women are turning to hypnobirthing as a natural technique for coping during labour. Women who are particularly frightened about giving birth may find it calming and relaxing. The idea is that mums-to-be and their birthing partners learn simple self-hypnosis, relaxation and breathing techniques – the aim of which is to have a better, calmer birth.

WHEN SHOULD I START LEARNING HYPNOBIRTHING TECHNIQUES?

The best time to start learning techniques – either by reading a hypnobirthing book, listening to a specialist hypnobirthing CD or attending a class – is said to be at the beginning of your third trimester. Classes can be quite expensive but you will learn skills including positions for labour and birth, breathing techniques, self-hypnosis and relaxation.

Decide where you'd like to give birth

Understand the different options – Depending on where you live in the UK, you may have been asked to make a decision on where you'd like to give birth right at the beginning of your pregnancy. Other mums-to-be aren't asked to confirm their decision until the third trimester. Providing that your pregnancy is classed as 'low risk', you may be able to choose where you would like to give birth – at hospital in a midwife-led unit or consultant-led unit. You may even want to give birth at home. If your pregnancy is complicated, you may not be able to choose to give birth anywhere but a consultant-led unit due to the extra medical support you may need. All expectant mothers have the right to ask for an elective caesarean but it's down to individual consultants to agree to this or not.

Write a birth plan

Think about how you'd like to give birth – With your due date edging closer, it's a good idea to start making decisions on your preference for giving birth – such as who you'd like as your birth partners (you can have two), the pain relief you'd ideally choose (choices may include gas and air, pethidine, epidural and water birth, but for more information see pages 143–144, Chapter 6). It can help to write this down in a birth plan, which you can print out to give to your midwife. It's a good idea to keep a copy of the plan in your handheld notes too.

Try not to have unrealistic expectations – If this is your first pregnancy and labour, it's difficult to imagine how it will really pan out. And, of course, nothing is certain. Many women find that the most painstakingly written birth plans go immediately out of the window once they're in labour. It can be helpful to have talked things through with your birth partner so that they can support you if things take an unexpected turn, such as if you need to have an emergency caesarean section due to unforeseen circumstances.

Practise safe, relaxing exercises and breathing techniques

Exercise in water to ease backache – As your due date nears, you may find that even short walks become tiring, particularly if your bump is large and you are suffering from shortness of breath – as many women do. Gentle water-based exercise is a great alternative because it supports the bump.

Relax through movement, as your due date approaches – Using movement can be an excellent way of encouraging relaxation. Try these two exercises from pregnancy and postnatal fitness expert, Dr Joanna Helcké.

Pelvic tilts and pelvic clock on a birthing ball

Joanna says: 'In late pregnancy it is very common to have all sorts of niggling aches and areas of tightness, especially in the lower back and pelvic area. These two gentle, rhythmic movements will help relieve tightness in the lower back all whilst being very relaxing. They are perfect for late pregnancy and the early stages of labour.'

1. Sit tall on a birthing ball (Swiss ball) with your feet firmly planted about shoulder width apart. Your hips should be higher than your knees when seated.

2. To get your posture perfect and ease away tension, focus on lengthening through the crown of your head, rolling your shoulders back so that your chest opens, and relaxing and dropping your shoulders down away from your ears.

3. To perform your pelvic tilts simply tuck the pelvis under, letting the ball roll forwards underneath you. You will feel a gentle stretch in your lower back as you tilt your pelvis backwards and forwards.

4. Keep going with this rhythmic rocking motion until your lower back feels mobile and any lightness has eased.

5. Now change your movement pattern to pelvic circles, making them as big or as small as feels comfortable and helpful. Let the ball roll under you as you push your hips forwards, out to the side, to the back, and then over to the other side. Remember to circle in both directions.

Learn about breathing techniques – If you've attended antenatal classes or pregnancy yoga, you'll have learnt about the benefits of breathing techniques as a way to relax you and conserve energy during labour.

During contractions, the pain can cause you to take quick, shallow breaths. This limits your oxygen intake, which can make you feel tired. Irregular breathing, along with feeling panicky and tense, can also stop the production of oxytocin – the hormone which helps your body deal naturally with labour. In contrast, taking deep regular breaths can make you feel relaxed and more focused. It may help you 'zone out' and lose track of the outside world as you focus on getting through your labour. Many women find it invaluable.

> **Tip**
>
> *Practise this simple breathing technique*
>
> ▶ Breathe in slowly through the nose, counting to three.
>
> ▶ Breathe out slowly through your mouth, again counting to three as you do it.
>
> ▶ Repeat this several times, getting used to the rhythm of your breathing.
>
> ▶ Ask your birthing partner to practise your breathing with you, before your due date, so that they're prepared to help you during labour.

Prepare your home

Prepare your home for the new arrival – You may already have repainted your home top to bottom, in the nesting stage. It can also be useful to stock up your kitchen cupboards and fill your freezer with some ready meals – or easy dishes such as lasagne and stews, which you can defrost for meals in the early days. Don't underestimate how little time you'll have for cooking meals in the first few weeks and you'll need to keep up your strength by eating well, especially if you're breastfeeding.

Prepare your baby's layette

Know what basics your baby will need – A 'layette' is the basic collection of clothes and bedding needed by your newborn in the first few weeks of life. Remember that the most important thing is for your baby to be warm and comfortable. Don't worry about elaborate outfits right now, even if it's really tempting to splurge!

Tip

Before you start shopping for your baby...

It's worth bearing in mind that friends and relatives will probably shower you with gifts of cute clothes, especially if this is your firstborn. So it's worth only buying the basics yourself. To save money, you can often find good quality second-hand baby clothes in charity shops, at NCT sales and on sites such as eBay and Gumtree. There may also be a local selling page in your area on Facebook. Always keep the tags in baby clothes and keep the receipts in case they are the wrong size and you need to take them back for an exchange or refund.

Basic layette

▶ Around six cotton long-sleeved babygrows with popper fastenings (choose size 0–3 months, as newborn sizes are tiny and most babies grow out of them very quickly. It's also a good idea to buy several, as newborns can get through several babygrows a day, if they're sick or produce a particularly leaky nappy!)

▶ Six cotton vests

▶ Bootees or baby socks (check inside for any loose threads, which should be removed)

- ▸ Scratch mittens

- ▸ Two or three cardigans

- ▸ Warm hat (for a winter baby) or a cotton jersey hat (for a summer baby)

- ▸ Warm jacket or snow-suit with warm bootees attached (if you have a winter baby)

- ▸ One or two soft cotton blankets

- ▸ Cotton sheets and blankets or a sleeping bag for baby's Moses basket or cot (duvets and pillows are not recommended until your baby's first birthday)

- ▸ Sheets and blanket for baby's pram or buggy

- ▸ Soft muslin squares (for mopping up spills but can also be used as an impromptu blanket, bib or even sunshade)

- ▸ Soft towels and flannels for bathtime.

Know about useful equipment for the first few weeks

Look into the baby equipment that will make your life easier – Here's a list for the first few months but do remember that 'what you need' is subjective. What one parent finds 'essential', another may never need to use. And bear in mind that you don't have to rush out and buy everything before your baby arrives. Shops (and online shopping) will still exist once your baby is here!

- ▸ Buggy – There are myriad options when it comes to buggies, prams and travel systems. Your best bet, when choosing, is to work out what you need your buggy to do (fit into tight spaces on buses and trains – or travel on rugged terrain) and then narrow down your search that way. The most important thing to remember is that it's suitable from birth, which means that your baby should be able to lie flat in it. Take care to check that whatever buggy you choose will fit in the boot of your car too! Some mums find that they don't need a buggy at all and manage by carrying their newborn around in a sling. But bear in mind that, if you've had a C-section or are suffering back pain following the delivery, using a sling in the first few weeks may not be possible.

▶ Car seat in newborn size   Make sure the make and model car seat you've chosen fits into your car securely.

▶ Moses basket, side nest, which can be attached to your bed or cot – Experts advise that new parents have their babies sleeping in the same room as them – day and night – for the first six months (see pages 153–154 for more information on safer sleeping). If you follow this advice, you may wish to have a portable Moses basket or carrycot, which you can move around your home for daytime naps.

▶ Bouncy chair – Somewhere safe to put your baby during the day, if you need your hands free for short periods of time.

▶ Breast pump (if you're planning on breastfeeding)

▶ Bottles (for formula feeding or for storing your expressed breast milk) plus bottlebrush and teat brush for cleaning

▶ Bottle steriliser (although boiling water in a pan is just as effective and a cheaper option!)

▶ A comfy chair for you to sit in for breastfeeding/bottle feeding – There are specific nursing chairs on the market but these are quite expensive and are in no way essential. Just make sure that you have a comfortable, supportive chair for you to sit in with your baby for extended periods of time.

▶ Breast pads

▶ Baby change mat

▶ Baby bath or bath support – Although you can feasibly bathe your baby in the bathroom sink, you may prefer a specifically designed plastic baby bath or a bath support to cradle baby so that you can wash them in the main bath.

▶ Cotton wool (for nappy changes)

▶ Nappies

▶ Nappy pail (if you're planning on using reusable nappies)

▶ Nappy bin (for disposable nappies)

▶ Barrier cream

▶ Room thermometer – It's important to keep an eye on the room temperature where your baby is sleeping; it should be between 16°C to 20°C (for more information on safe sleeping, see pages 153–154).

▶ A basic first aid kit containing saline nasal drops, digital thermometer, liquid pain relief and an oral syringe

Be savvy with your cash – You don't have to spend a fortune on baby equipment (unless you want to!). Second-hand bargains can be found online or at NCT sales or you may be given equipment by family and friends.

> ⚠ **WARNING**
>
> There are certain items that should always be bought new. They are:
>
> **Car seat** – If you buy a second-hand car seat, you have no way of knowing whether it's been involved in an accident, during which it may have been damaged.
>
> **Cot/Moses basket mattress** – If you're using a second-hand cot or Moses basket, you should always buy a new mattress. Second-hand mattresses may not have been stored in a dry environment. This could cause mould spores to develop within the fibres of the mattress. Research has found that the use of second-hand cot mattresses can increase the risk of cot death.

If you're planning a home birth, be prepared

Know the facts about home births – If you are healthy and your pregnancy is considered low risk, you can choose the option of a home birth. However, it's important to be realistic. More women want a home birth than actually end up having one, due to complications which may develop during labour, such as the baby becoming distressed or the labour not progressing. A home birthing mum requiring an epidural (when anaesthetic drugs are passed into the small of the back via a fine tube, to numb that area of the body) will also be taken to hospital, as an anaesthetist can only administer this. Also, if you decide that you want to go into hospital or to a birthing centre partway through your labour at home, your midwife can arrange for you to be transferred. It's thought that around one-fifth of women, with low-risk pregnancies who embark on a home birth, are transferred to hospital to deliver their baby.

WHO WILL BE THERE AT A HOME BIRTH?

Ideally, you'll have two community midwives with you when your baby is being born – although they may not both be there during your entire labour. What usually happens is that one midwife will visit during your labour, to check how you're coping. Then the second midwife will arrive as you are preparing to deliver. It's also important to choose a birthing partner who can support you during your home birth.

Be prepared for your home birth – A few weeks before your due date, your midwife will bring you a birth pack, containing essentials that she'll need during the birth. You may also want to have the following items prepared:

- ▶ Plastic sheeting and towels to protect the area where you are planning on delivering – your carpet or bed

- ▶ A blanket in case you get cold

- ▶ Bin liners for rubbish

▶ A birthing pool, if you're planning a water birth (these can be bought new or second-hand or hired – ask your midwife for advice)

▶ Clean towels and a blanket for your baby after the birth

▶ You'll also need all the items you'd take to hospital (see section below).

Or prepare for your hospital birth

Pack your hospital bag – If you're planning on giving birth in hospital, it's advisable to have a bag packed from around 36 weeks. But it can be difficult to know what to pack for hospital, when you don't know how long you'll be staying. Here's a guide to the basics:

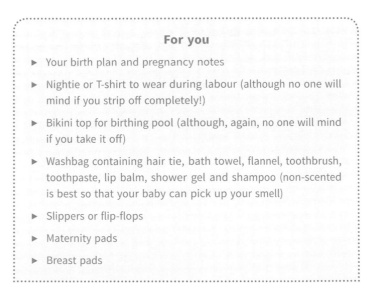

For you

▶ Your birth plan and pregnancy notes

▶ Nightie or T-shirt to wear during labour (although no one will mind if you strip off completely!)

▶ Bikini top for birthing pool (although, again, no one will mind if you take it off)

▶ Washbag containing hair tie, bath towel, flannel, toothbrush, toothpaste, lip balm, shower gel and shampoo (non-scented is best so that your baby can pick up your smell)

▶ Slippers or flip-flops

▶ Maternity pads

▶ Breast pads

- ► Fresh nightie for wearing after birth
- ► Clean, comfortable clothes for travelling home
- ► Comfortable knickers and thick socks (many women find their feet get very cold in labour)
- ► Two nursing bras
- ► Pillow
- ► Light blanket
- ► Small change for snacks/drinks
- ► Snacks and drinks for labour
- ► Magazines and books, in case it takes a while
- ► Ice cubes to suck (keep them in a vacuum flask)
- ► Music to listen to during labour – Check beforehand whether there are CD players or iPod docks in labour rooms.

For baby

- ► Nappies – around 20 in newborn size
- ► Cotton wool (for nappy changes and cleaning your baby's skin – experts advise against baby wipes, lotions, shampoo and talc for the first six weeks and to only use water for cleaning)
- ► Two baby vests
- ► Scratch mittens
- ► Two long-sleeved babygrows
- ► Socks
- ► Muslin squares

▶ Cardigan, blanket and hat for the journey home – and a winter suit if you're having a winter baby.

REMEMBER that if you're taking your baby home by car, you must have a car seat, which should be fitted correctly. Many first-time parents struggle to fit the car seat when it comes to leaving the hospital with their precious cargo. So it's a good idea for you or your partner to have practised fitting it before you go into labour to avoid any last-minute panics on the big day. Remember: A rear-facing car seat **must not** be placed in a seat protected by an active frontal airbag because it can cause serious injury or death to the child.

For birthing partner

▶ Comfortable clothing and footwear – T-shirts are best as labour rooms are warm

▶ Extra T-shirt and a washbag with flannel, face wipes, toothbrush and toothpaste – in case they end up staying a while

▶ Swimwear and a towel (if accompanying partner in birthing pool)

▶ Cash for car parking, snacks and drinks from hospital canteen/vending machine

▶ Snacks from home if preferred

▶ Book or magazine (in case things take a while)

▶ Camera/video camera

▶ Fully charged mobile phone and charger – Your birth partner should act as the main point of contact for relatives so that you don't have to worry about making calls or sending texts.

Be prepared for whatever your labour and birth experience will bring – Whether this will be your first experience of giving birth or not, it's good to be prepared for what may happen. (If you are having a planned caesarean section, your doctor will guide you through the process in the weeks approaching your selected delivery date.)

Know about going overdue and inductions

Don't be surprised if you go overdue – Most babies arrive between 37 and 41 weeks of pregnancy (NHS 2010, NHS 2011a). If you sail past your due date without a twinge, it can be frustrating, especially if you're fielding well-meaning calls and texts from family and friends. Remember that going 'overdue' is not a sign of failure.

Know about the possible ways of kick-starting labour – Your midwife may offer you a cervical sweep to try to get things going. There are also some 'natural' ways, which some people believe can start contractions – but you should take these with a large pinch of salt. They include: having sex, eating a hot curry and eating the heart of a pineapple! Some mums-to-be like to bounce on a birthing ball in an attempt to start contractions, while others drink raspberry leaf tea. The truth is that your baby will come when it's ready.

Know about inductions – You won't be allowed to go more than two weeks overdue, due to the potential risk to your baby. So you may be scheduled for a hospital induction in this instance, which means that you'll be given intravenous drugs in order to start labour. Inductions can cause rapid, intense contractions, which can be a real shock to your system. Rest assured that this is normal and make sure that your midwife or doctor has talked through your pain relief options (see below) with you beforehand so that you are prepared.

Be clued up about pain relief options during labour – The reality is that labour can hurt – although different women seem to experience it to different degrees. But the prospect of dealing with pain can be frightening for many. However, there are a number of methods of helping you through the pain of contractions and giving birth. One thing to remember is that giving birth is not a competition and, despite what some people may tell you, you won't receive a gold medal for giving birth without any pain relief. The most important thing is that your baby is born safely and that your wellbeing is looked after at all times too. Below are some of the options you might want to consider:

▶ Hypnobirthing (see page 128)

▶ Breathing techniques (see pages 131–132)

▶ TENS machine – A handheld controller connected by leads to four sticky pads placed on your back. It gives out tiny pulses of electrical energy, which give a tingling sensation on the skin and can help distract from the pain of contractions, especially during early labour. You can buy these new or hire them for the birth.

▶ Water pool – Many women opt for water births these days because warm water is relaxing and can ease the pain of contractions. The water is kept no warmer than 37.5 °C and your temperature is monitored throughout. You should check whether your hospital has a water pool available, if you think that you'd like to choose this option. For home births, you can buy or hire specialist pools.

► Gas and air (entonox) – A combination of oxygen and nitrous oxide gas, it won't take away all the pain but it can make it more bearable. You take deep breaths of the gas and air through a handheld mouthpiece. The gas takes around 15 to 20 seconds to work and you breathe it in as a contraction begins. There are no side effects but it can make you feel light-headed, which can help take the edge off things! It can also be used in a water pool.

► Epidural – A local anaesthetic fed into your back through a fine tube, which numbs the whole area around your back and tummy and may also make your legs feel immobile and heavy, which means that you will have to stay in one position rather than being able to move around the room or sit in a water pool. It is usually used in particularly long, complicated or painful labours and offers complete pain relief. It can only be administered by an anaesthetist and so is not available during home births or in a water pool.

► Pethidine – An injection into the muscle in your thigh or buttock of the drug pethidine can lessen the pain and help you relax. The effects last up to four hours so it cannot be used in a water pool. It can also make some women feel sick and can make it difficult to push. If the drug passes to your baby during labour, it may affect their breathing and their first feed.

Be prepared for early labour, including recognising the signs and coping with contractions

Recognise the signs that you're approaching labour – You'll probably get a 'show', which is when the mucus plug comes away from your cervix. It may come out when you go to the toilet and can happen a few days before or immediately before you go into labour.

Know when you're in labour – You may get strong regular contractions, your waters may break, you may feel an urgent need to go to the toilet or suddenly experience strong backache.

Know what to do if your waters break without signs of contractions starting – If your waters break but you aren't experiencing contractions, call the hospital. You may be asked to go in for monitoring. If your contractions don't start after a certain time, you may be induced to avoid the risk of infection.

Know whether you're having contractions or not – In your last weeks of pregnancy, you'll probably experience Braxton Hicks (discussed on page 114, Chapter 5), which are thought to be a sign of your uterus tightening and then relaxing in preparation for birth. Actual contractions, which mean that you're in labour, feel different. Some women describe them as being like period pains, which last longer than 30 seconds and gradually get more painful and frequent.

Note the timings – It can be helpful to mark down the timings of these contractions in order to note how frequently they are coming. It might be easier for your birthing partner to do this as this stage can last for several hours.

Know about pain relief in early labour – If you're labouring at home in the early stages, you could try a number of different pain relief tactics including:

▶ using a TENS machine

▶ taking paracetamol

▶ using a hot water bottle against your back, if you have back pain

▶ bouncing or resting on a birthing ball

▶ sitting in a warm bath or shower

▶ massage from your partner

▶ breathing techniques (which you may have learnt about at antenatal classes or from your midwife – see also pages 131– 132)

▶ hypnobirthing techniques (if you've practised them)

Know when to go to hospital and what happens there

Get the timing right – If you are intending on giving birth in hospital, most ask you not to go to the maternity unit until either your waters have broken or your contractions are lasting around

50–60 seconds and are coming around every five minutes. But if you are at all unsure, call the hospital and ask to speak to a midwife. Not all 'active' labour pains fit the criteria of contraction timings. A midwife can often tell how far along you are by 'listening' to a contraction and speaking to you. If you have decided to set off to hospital, call them to tell them that you're on your way. If you are hoping for a water birth, don't forget to tell them this when you call so that they can prepare a pool if one is available.

Be prepared for what will happen when you get to hospital – Once you've arrived, you should hand your notes to the admissions desk. A midwife will take you to a private room to examine you to ensure that you're far enough along to be admitted (if you go too early, before your contractions are coming every five minutes, bear in mind that you may be sent home again). They'll also check your blood pressure, your temperature and your pulse and check your urine. They'll listen to your baby's heartbeat and feel your abdomen to check the baby's position. They'll probably also do an internal examination to see how far your cervix has opened – to determine how far labour has progressed.

These checks will be repeated throughout your labour. It's important you ask questions, if you feel you need to. And, if you have a birth plan, show it to the midwife.

You'll be taken to a delivery room where you can get changed into something light and comfortable for giving birth. If you've requested a birthing pool and it's available, you can get into the water. Delivery rooms usually have an en suite bathroom where you can have a bath or shower, if you would like to. There may be a TV and a CD player. It's important that you and your birthing partner feel comfortable in the delivery room.

Be clear about pain relief – You will have a choice of pain relief. You may want gas and air or if you are on a consultant-led ward, you may have requested an epidural. If you're using a TENS machine you may want to continue with this or use your breathing techniques. As your labour progresses, your preference for pain relief may alter.

Know about the three stages of labour

Know about the three stages of labour – The process of giving birth can be divided into three sections:

First stage – Contractions cause your cervix to dilate (open). This is the longest stage and can take several hours.

Second stage – Once your cervix is dilated 10 cm (fully open), you can start pushing your baby through your vagina with your contractions. At this stage, most women feel an urge to push.

If there are no complications, you should be able to deliver your baby naturally. But in some instances, if the baby is in an awkward position such as back to back (when your baby is lying with its back against your back), you may require assistance from doctors in the form of a ventouse or forceps delivery. You may also require an episiotomy – a cut to the perineum and posterior vaginal wall in order to allow the baby to be delivered (see page 115, Chapter 5).

If your midwife or doctor feels that it would be safer to deliver your baby by emergency caesarean (if your baby is in distress or if you are thought to be at risk), the decision may be taken to prep you for surgery. You and your birth partner will be kept informed and should be talked through this procedure.

Third stage – After your baby has been delivered and the umbilical cord has been clamped, you will deliver the placenta. This can happen in two ways: naturally or managed – and you may be able to choose your preferred way (although sometimes circumstance determines what happens). Naturally means waiting for your womb to contract, causing you to push out the placenta. Managed means that you are given an injection of a drug (ergometrine) in your thigh. The cord will be clamped to avoid the drug being passed to your baby. The injection encourages a contraction, causing your placenta to come away from the wall of your womb. The midwife may then encourage you to push out the placenta or she can pull it out for you. If you've had an episiotomy or have torn, you'll be stitched up. You shouldn't feel any of this, as you'll be given a local anaesthetic injection and you can also request gas and air (see page 114) should you need it.

Know what to expect when your baby arrives

Get ready for your first cuddle – The moment is finally here. Once your newborn has been delivered and checked over, they will be handed to you. Skin-to-skin contact is encouraged, so your little one will be placed against your naked chest for that all-important first cuddle and feed (if you've chosen to breastfeed). Make sure your birthing partner has the camera ready to snap some precious first pics!

Understand it might take some time – People often wax lyrical about the immediate 'rush of love' new mums feel when they hold their newborn for the first time. For many women, this is absolutely the case. But, depending on your birth experience, you may feel a mix of shock and exhaustion too. Some women even report feeling emotionally detached as they hold this new little person in their arms for the first time. If this happens to you, try not to beat yourself up emotionally and accept that sometimes the bonding process takes a little time. Some women find that their maternal love suddenly appears, in overpowering form, a little later on once their emotions have settled down. It doesn't mean you are any less of a mother at all.

Know about colostrum – Even if you choose not to breastfeed long term, just feeding your baby for their first few days provides them with colostrum – the milky fluid that comes before the true milk appears. It contains carbohydrates, fats, vitamins, minerals and proteins (antibodies), which fight disease-causing agents such as bacteria and viruses. It's such a benefit to your baby if you can give them this.

Know about the vitamin K injection – Before giving birth, you should already have been given information about the vitamin K injection. Vitamin K is essential to stop bleeding but some babies aren't born with enough in their system, which means that their blood may not clot. The vitamin K injection will be offered to your baby in the first 24 hours of their life. You need to give your permission for your baby to have it.

Be prepared to stay overnight in hospital – Depending on whether you've had a straightforward birth or there have been complications, such as intervention including a ventouse, forceps or emergency caesarean delivery, you may need to stay in hospital overnight or longer. You will be transferred to the postnatal ward after giving birth, along with your baby (unless they have been born with health issues, in which case they may be taken to the neonatal unit for specialist care and you will be kept informed of their treatment at all times).

Know what to expect from the postnatal ward – Here, you should be given support and advice on feeding and caring for your baby. If you have any questions, don't be afraid to ask the midwives and nurses on the ward. You will also be monitored. Be aware that you will lose blood from your vagina post birth (this is called lochia) so you should wear maternity pads and change them regularly. If you've had stitches – from an episiotomy or caesarean – these will be checked regularly. You may be given help to have your first shower or bath on the postnatal ward. If you are having any issues with breastfeeding, a breastfeeding consultant may come to see you and offer advice. Make sure you have something light to wear in the postnatal ward as the heating tends to be cranked up quite high for the babies' benefit.

Decide whether you'd like visitors or not – Most postnatal wards allow visitors at restricted times. You may well want to show off your newborn as soon as possible but remember that it's your decision whether you have visitors in hospital or whether to wait until you and your baby are safely home. Make sure that you are clear in your wishes so that people don't turn up unannounced – and uninvited – to hospital.

Going home – Once your baby has passed his or her newborn checks and you are also deemed fit to leave hospital, you can prepare to leave. Remember that, if you are leaving by car, the hospital requires you to take your baby home in a car seat, which should be fitted correctly.

Be prepared for the early days

Settling in back home – The first few days and weeks with your newborn can be a magical time. But don't be surprised if you find yourself experiencing a rollercoaster of emotions. Lots of new mums experience the baby blues a few days after giving birth, when they may feel particularly tearful and emotional. This usually ties in with their milk coming in. Sleep deprivation can also make you feel very unsettled. Be honest about your feelings and don't be afraid to admit that you are overwhelmed.

If you can't shake off the baby blues, seek help – Don't be afraid to tell your midwife (who will visit you in the early days) or your health visitor (who will take over from your midwife after the first week or so), if you can't seem to shake your sadness. Unfortunately, many new mums do go through postnatal depression and there is help available.

Be clear about visitors in the early days – Many new parents find themselves swamped with people 'popping in' when the last thing they want to do is to entertain. So, if you'd prefer to be left alone for the first few days, that's perfectly acceptable.

Be aware of safe sleeping methods – Follow this guide to reduce the risk of SIDS (sudden infant death syndrome) – formerly known as cot death. For more guidance go to www.lullabytrust.org.uk/safer-sleep.

► Official guidelines state that babies are safest sleeping – day or night – in the same room as you for the first six months. So you may wish to move your baby's carrycot or Moses basket around your home for daytime naps, so that you can always see them.

► Always place your baby on their back to sleep with their feet at the end of the cot or pram (to stop them wriggling down under their blanket).

► Use a firm, flat, waterproof mattress.

► Keep the room temperature where your baby is sleeping between 16 °C and 20 °C.

► Don't share a bed with your baby, if either you or your partner has been drinking alcohol, taking drugs or smoking, if you are extremely tired, or if your baby was of low birth weight or born prematurely.

▶ Never go to sleep holding your baby whilst sitting in an armchair or on a sofa.

▶ Don't allow your baby to get too hot – remove hats when they're sleeping and make sure their blanket is no higher than their shoulders.

▶ Remove all soft bedding, cot bumpers, pillows and soft toys from your baby's cot to avoid accidents.

Do what is right for you and your family – Just like during pregnancy, people will be keen to give you advice on sleeping routines, on feeding and even on how to dress your baby! Some advice can be helpful but feel free to take most of it with a pinch of salt. Remember, this is YOUR baby and YOUR family. Ask for support and help but remember that any decisions are yours and your partner's to make. All being well, this is the start of a wonderful journey together… good luck!

Quotes from experts

BIRTH PLAN

❝ It's important to write a birth plan but even more vital to research the issues that are on it. What happens to women in childbirth can have a lifelong physical and psychological impact so ensure the choices you make are informed ones and know your rights. ❞

Virginia Howes, midwife

Quotes from parents and parents-to-be

ANTENATAL CLASSES

❝ The friends I made through NCT have been invaluable. Nobody else cares SO much about poo and sleep. We've kept each other sane throughout this first year. ❞

Susie, mum to Bridget, 13 months

❝ We decided to do antenatal classes. We'd just relocated to a new area and thought it was a good way to meet people. My partner didn't mind the main part of the classes but absolutely hated the relaxation bit at the end. ❞

Andreina, mum to Rufus, 17 months

COPING WITH LABOUR

❝ I laughed when my midwife recommended that I bake a cake during the early stages of labour. But 17 hours into my contractions, I started to bake and it was brilliant. It kept me 'active', killed time and when we came back from the hospital the next day we had an extra special chocolate cake to share with our families over a cup of tea. **❞**

Susie, mum to Bridget, 13 months

DAD'S VIEWPOINT

❝ As my wife's due date neared, I worried most about how I'd be able to help her during labour and what practical things I could do. We talked it all through before the birth and it turned out that we worked really well as a team. **❞**

Chris, dad to Marianne, three years

CHAPTER 7
POSSIBLE HEALTH PROBLEMS DURING PREGNANCY

Be clued up about potential problems

Most women generally have an enjoyable and problem-free pregnancy. Hopefully you'll be one of them! But it's important to be aware about potential health problems. That way you can recognise any symptoms in yourself and get them checked out promptly.

Here's a glossary, in alphabetical order, of the most common health issues that may arise during pregnancy. Remember that if you have any health concerns during your pregnancy, your best bet is to consult a medical professional as soon as possible.

Backache is common during pregnancy, especially during the second and third trimesters. This is because your ligaments become softer and stretch to prepare for labour. It can put a strain on your lower back and pelvis. To help avoid backache, try to do exercises to strengthen your abdominal muscles, as this supports your back (see the exercise on page 99, Chapter 4). You should also avoid carrying heavy objects, bend your knees and keep your back straight when lifting something off the ground, sleep on a firm mattress and make sure you get plenty of rest. Pregnancy massage may also help ease back pain.

Bleeding – It can be quite common to have light bleeding or 'spotting' during the first weeks of pregnancy, especially around the time that your period would be due. It's always a good idea to mention it to your midwife if it happens to you. Seek medical help immediately if you experience heavy bleeding or if stomach pains accompany any bleeding.

Carpal tunnel syndrome is a condition that causes numbness, tingling, pain or a dull ache in the fingers, hands or wrists. It is extremely common in pregnancy and tends to appear in the second half of pregnancy when women tend to retain more fluid, causing pressure to press on the carpal tunnel nerve. You can help yourself during pregnancy by avoiding activities such as typing, which may aggravate symptoms, and wearing a wrist or hand brace. Symptoms usually disappear after giving birth.

Ectopic pregnancy happens when a fertilised egg implants itself outside the womb, usually in a fallopian tube. This can result in damage to the fallopian tube and can cause life-threatening bleeding. Signs of a ruptured fallopian tube are severe, acute pain, dizziness, sickness, shoulder pain and diarrhoea. If you think this is happening to you, you should seek immediate medical help at hospital.

Gestational diabetes is a type of diabetes that develops during pregnancy, usually in the third trimester. It's caused when women have higher than normal levels of glucose, which their body can't bring under control with insulin. All women are tested for it during pregnancy. Symptoms include a dry mouth with increased thirst, the need to urinate more frequently, blurred vision and tiredness. If not treated, it can cause birth complications but it generally disappears after giving birth. The condition can be controlled with diet and exercise but some women require medication.

Headaches are common in pregnancy, especially in the first trimester. This is thought to be due to raging hormones, lack of sleep and sometimes dehydration so try to drink plenty of fluids. Massage and acupuncture can help and paracetamol is considered safe to take during pregnancy too (although the Royal College of Midwives advises that you check with your midwife or GP before taking it). Occasionally, in later trimesters, severe headaches can be a sign of something serious, such as pre-eclampsia. If you have a strong headache for the first time in late pregnancy, contact your GP or midwife so that you can be checked over.

Hyperemesis gravidarum is extreme pregnancy sickness, thought to affect one in every 100 women. It can cause sufferers to vomit up to 50 times a day, making it impossible to keep fluids and food down. It's a debilitating condition that can lead to serious complications including malnourishment, dehydration, ketosis, serious weight loss and low blood pressure. If you're drinking less than 500 ml of fluid a day and have lost weight during the first weeks of your pregnancy, you must seek help. Sufferers may be prescribed anti-sickness medication and, if vomiting cannot be controlled, may be admitted to hospital for intravenous treatment (drugs given directly through a drip).

Itchy skin is thought to affect a quarter of pregnant women. For most, it's more annoying than a sign of serious problems. It could be due to stretching skin or changing hormones and may mainly affect your breasts and bump. Skin complaints such as eczema could also be to blame and some women experience eczema for the first time during pregnancy. Your GP can prescribe treatments to soothe eczema. Thrush or scabies could also be to blame – again, your GP can help. In some instances, severe and prolonged itching can be a sign of a liver problem so you should always mention it your doctor or midwife.

Iron-deficiency anaemia affects almost a quarter of women in the UK during pregnancy. You need 14.8 mg of iron every day when you're pregnant. This is to keep oxygen pumping to your vital organs through your blood – and to keep your baby healthy. If a blood test finds that your iron levels are lacking, your midwife may prescribe iron supplements to boost them. You can also boost your iron levels further with iron-rich foods including red meat, poultry and fish, dried fruit, fortified cereals (check the label), pulses, green leafy vegetables and wholegrain bread.

Leg cramps may strike during your second and third trimesters, especially at night when you're in bed. As your bump gets heavier, your legs will take much of the strain during the day. Also, your growing uterus puts pressure on the main vein from your legs, which can spark the pains. Leg cramps may also be a sign that you're lacking salts and nutrients so you could take a pregnancy supplement containing magnesium. Keeping your legs slightly elevated in bed, by resting them on a pillow, can help. To ease a cramp, straighten your leg, heel first, and flex your toes and ankles – or massage the muscle. Alternatively, you could get out of bed and walk around until the pain goes.

Obstetric cholestasis is a rare pregnancy condition of the liver, which can develop in the third trimester due to a build of bile acids in the bloodstream. It can cause severe skin itching but symptoms usually disappear after delivery. There is a tiny chance it could lead to complications during birth so affected women need to be monitored.

Pica is a rare condition that affects a tiny number of women for the first time during pregnancy. It causes them to crave substances with little or no nutritional value, such as coal, glue or even carpet. The word pica is Latin for magpie – a bird famous for eating almost anything. No one knows the cause but some experts believe that the cravings are a sign of something missing in the diet, such as iron or essential vitamins. It goes without saying that eating substances such as carpet could cause you – and your unborn child – serious harm and you should speak to your GP if you're affected.

Piles (or haemorrhoids) are swollen veins around the anus. During pregnancy, hormones, which make your veins relax, can cause piles to form. If you're affected, you may notice that they itch or feel sore, especially when you go to the toilet. You may be able to feel them as small lumps around your anus and they may bleed slightly. Constipation can also cause piles. You can ease piles by eating a diet high in fibre and staying hydrated to ease constipation. Regular exercise can also help. Your GP may prescribe safe medicines or creams to ease pain. Most piles disappear within weeks of birth.

Polyhydramnios is a common complication which means that there's too much amniotic fluid surrounding your unborn baby. It is usually detected after 30 weeks. It sometimes indicates a problem with the baby's development, such as a blockage in their gut. But most women with the condition have healthy babies. One telltale sign to look out for includes your belly getting big very quickly. Although the cause is not known, it can be linked with women who have diabetes, or rhesus disease, as well as women pregnant with twins.

Pre-eclampsia is a serious condition affecting some women in the second half of pregnancy (after 20 weeks or soon after giving birth). Early signs include high blood pressure and protein in the urine. This is why you should have your blood pressure and your urine checked during every antenatal appointment. Other symptoms include severe headache, vision problems and fluid retention, which cause swelling of the ankles, hands and feet. If you develop any of these symptoms, you should seek medical help immediately.

Premature birth is the birth of a baby at less than full term (37 weeks). There can be a number of causes for a woman to have a premature baby, including diabetes and high blood pressure. Some babies have survived after being born at 24 weeks, thanks to advances in medical care for premature babies, who are usually cared for in specialist hospital neonatal units. But there is an increased risk of long-term health issues and disabilities when a baby is born very early.

Pre-term premature rupture of membranes (PPROM) is a rare occurrence when the mother's waters break very early – before their baby has reached full term. If your waters break before 37 weeks, it means that the amniotic fluid has leaked from the sac containing your baby. If this happens, you should seek immediate medical help as both your baby and you could be at risk of serious infection.

Restless leg syndrome (RLS) is a condition which can strike in pregnancy, peaking at around seven or eight months pregnant. It causes sufferers to feel an uncontrollable urge to move their legs to relieve a tingling or burning sensation. It is often worse at night and can also affect the hands and arms. The cause isn't known but thankfully it's temporary and usually disappears within a month of giving birth.

Symphysis pubis dysfunction (SPD) or pelvic girdle pain is thought to affect one in four pregnant women, in varying degrees of severity. It can start from any time towards the end of the first trimester. It's caused by the ligaments softening in your pelvis to prepare for birth, which causes the pelvic joints to move more, leading to pain and inflammation. If you are diagnosed with SPD, your GP or midwife can refer you to a physiotherapist.

Thrush is a yeast infection in the vagina, which causes itching and discomfort. It's fairly common in pregnancy, due to hormone changes. Your GP can prescribe pregnancy-safe antifungal pessaries and creams that are suitable for your stage of pregnancy.

Varicose veins are veins that have become swollen and twisted and may appear blue or purple, usually on the legs. They develop when small valves inside the veins stop working, causing blood to flow backwards and collect. One in three people suffer from them and pregnancy can increase the chance of them developing. This is because the weight of the uterus creates pressure on your veins. Lower your risk by avoiding sitting or standing still for extended periods, taking regular breaks and raising your legs when resting. Exercise can help by improving blood circulation. Varicose veins usually disappear after pregnancy but some women need treatment.

WHAT IF SOMETHING GOES WRONG?

Coping with miscarriage – Although most pregnancies result in a happy, healthy baby, sadly there are some instances when this doesn't happen. If you're unlucky enough to lose your baby during any stage of your pregnancy, or have a stillbirth, it's important that you and your family have the support you need in this devastating time. If you have a later miscarriage, you can choose to have a memorial, burial or cremation. Stillbirths must be formally registered but this is not required with a miscarriage. But some hospitals can provide a certificate if you wish. Your GP should be able to guide you and arrange bereavement counselling, if you feel that it would help. You can also find advice and support at www.miscarriageassociation.org.uk.

There's no doubt that suffering a miscarriage or stillbirth is a horrendous experience. You may feel as though you'll never recover, emotionally. But please take heart and remember that it does not affect your chances of becoming pregnant again and going on to have a healthy baby in the future.

Many thanks to Liat for her help, to all those at Summersdale who put their trust in me to write this book, and to Sandy, who made the copy-editing process run smoothly.

Thank you to my very understanding husband, Chris, to my ever supportive parents, Jane and John, and to the rest of our brilliant family for their encouragement. Most of all, this is for Smithlet and Smithie, who've taught me (nearly) everything I need to know about pregnancy.

Thanks also to the wonderful parents and parents-to-be who kindly shared their experiences – and helpful tips – for this book.

ACKNOWLEDGEMENTS

With sincere thanks to the following medical experts, who have given valuable advice during the writing of this book.

Dr Joanna Helcké, pregnancy and postnatal fitness expert: www.joannahelcke.com

Dr Toni Hazell, MRCGP: www.tonihazell.co.uk

Virginia Howes RM, Bsc (Hons), independent midwife and author of *The Baby's Coming*

Dr Sarah Jarvis, clinical consultant at Patient: www.Patient.info

Dr Ruth Miller MPSNI, MRPharmS

Denise Knowles, relationship counsellor, Relate, which provides impartial relationship support including support when preparing for and adjusting to the arrival of a new baby: www.relate.org.uk

Elizabeth Hutton, CEO of Count the Kicks, pregnancy and stillbirth awareness charity: www.countthekicks.org.uk

Sally Wisbey, nutritional therapist (diploma in nutritional therapy and winner of the CAM 2014 award – 'highly commended for outstanding practice'): www.sallywisbeynutrition.co.uk

We have been careful to ensure that all the information in this book corresponds to the guidance given on the NHS Choices website. For information on the latest official pregnancy guidelines, visit www.nhs.uk.

INDEX

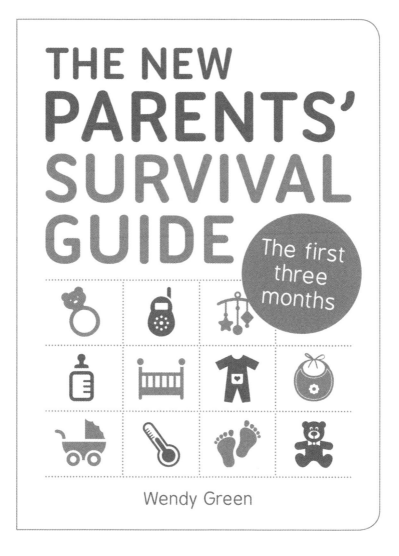

THE NEW PARENTS' SURVIVAL GUIDE

The first three months

Wendy Green

THE NEW PARENTS' SURVIVAL GUIDE
The First Three Months

Wendy Green

£7.99

Paperback

ISBN: 978-1-84953-715-5

Everything you need to know to guide you through your baby's first three months and beyond!

No matter how much you long for and plan for a baby, no one is quite prepared for the impact their new arrival has on their life. This book recognises that no one has a textbook-perfect baby and lets you in on what you can REALLY expect in the first three months. *The New Parents' Survival Guide* is packed with practical advice and simple tips on how to deal with common problems you are likely to encounter, including how to:

- Care for your newborn • Solve the breast versus bottle dilemma
- Overcome breastfeeding woes • Calm your crying baby
- Solve sleep issues • Manage minor ailments
- Take good care of yourself

NEW Old-Fashioned Parenting

A GUIDE TO HELP YOU FIND THE BALANCE
BETWEEN TRADITIONAL AND MODERN PARENTING

LIAT HUGHES JOSHI

NEW OLD-FASHIONED PARENTING

A Guide to Help You Find the Balance between Traditional and Modern Parenting

Liat Hughes Joshi

£10.99

Paperback

ISBN: 978-1-84953-672-1

There's been a revolution in the family; it's now all about the kids.

We've moved on from children being 'seen and not heard', but we're now plagued with the worry of ending up with 'that child' – the one who's running amok and is ill-prepared for life.

This book combines contemporary and traditional childrearing methods, bringing fresh thinking to some of the essential parenting issues of our time:

• Managing screen use • Encouraging independence
• Finding the balance between school and play • Compromising between parenting that's pushy and not involved enough • Establishing the 'best of both worlds' approach that works in the modern world for modern families.

In this manifesto of new old-fashioned parenting, there's no pandering, no spoiling, and definitely no dinosaur-shaped chicken nuggets at dinner time.

'The antidote to over-indulgent modern parenting. Challenges some of the ways we've come to think about what's best for our children and provides fresh, practical advice about parenting dilemmas of our times.'

Oliver James, psychologist and author of
Affluenza and *How Not to F*** Them Up*

Have you enjoyed this book?
If so, why not write a review on your favourite website?

If you're interested in finding out more about our books,
find us on Facebook at **Summersdale Publishers** and
follow us on Twitter at **@Summersdale**.

Thanks very much for buying this Summersdale book.

www.summersdale.com